Examination
of the Cranial
and Peripheral Nerves

Examination of the Cranial and Peripheral Nerves

Orrin Devinsky, M.D.

Medical Neurology Branch
National Institute of Neurological and
    Communicative Disorders and Stroke
National Institutes of Health
Bethesda, Maryland

Edward Feldmann, M.D.

Department of Neurology
New York Hospital-Cornell Medical Center
New York, New York

Elizabeth Beemster, Illustrator

Churchill Livingstone
New York, Edinburgh, London, Melbourne   1988

Library of Congress Cataloging in Publication Data

Devinsky, Orrin.
    Examination of the cranial and peripheral nerves / Orrin Devinsky,
Edward Feldmann ; Elizabeth Beemster, illustrator.
    p. cm.
    Includes bibliographies and index.
    ISBN 0-443-08562-5
    1. Nerves, Peripheral—Examination—Handbooks, manuals, etc. 2.
Nerves, Peripheral—Anatomy—Handbooks, manuals, etc. 3. Nerves,
Peripheral—Diseases—Diagnosis—Handbooks, manuals, etc. 4.
Nerves, Cranial—Examination—Handbooks, manuals, etc. 5. Nerves,
Cranial—Anatomy—Handbooks, manuals, etc. 6. Nerves, Cranial—
Diseases—Diagnosis—Handbooks, manuals, etc.
I. Feldmann, Edward. II. Title.
    [DNLM: 1. Cranial Nerves—handbooks. 2. Peripheral Nerves—
handbooks. WL 39 D495e]
RC409.D48 1988
616.8'7075—dc 19
DNLM/DLC
for Library of Congress   87-27841
                                              CIP

© **Churchill Livingstone Inc. 1988**

Distributed in the United Kingdom by Churchill Livingstone, Robert
Stevenson House, 1–3 Baxter's Place, Leith Walk, Edinburgh EH1
3AF, and by associated companies, branches, and representatives
throughout the world.

Accurate indications, adverse reactions, and dosage schedules for
drugs are provided in this book, but it is possible that they may
change. The reader is urged to review the package information data
of the manufacturers of the medications mentioned.

The opinions and assertions contained herein are the private views
of the authors, and are not to be construed as official or necessarily
reflecting the views of the National Institutes of Health.

Acquisitions Editor: *Beth Kaufman Barry*
Copy Editor: *Margot Otway*
Production Designer: *Gloria Brown*
Production Supervisor: *Jocelyn Eckstein*

Printed in the United States of America

First published in 1988

FOREWORD

Drs. Devinsky and Feldmann have concluded from their experience as neurological trainees that no fully satisfactory, succinct, and portable manual for the evaluation of peripheral nerve function presently exists. Accordingly, they have carefully synthesized this practical, direct, and highly useful pocket-sized handbook from various sources, some only brief in their previous presentation elsewhere, and some available only informally through training manuals of the Department of Neurology at New York Hospital-Cornell Medical Center. The volume should prove valuable to students and practitioners of medicine at every level and especially to neurologists, neurosurgeons, orthopaedists, physiatrists, and rehabilitation therapists, who constantly face the complexity of peripheral nerve diagnosis but have no quick, accurate, and clinically complete reference source at their fingertips. This guidebook, with its clear illustrations and useful didactic descriptions, should enjoy wide use and a long life.

Fred Plum, M.D.
Anne Parrish Titzell Professor of Neurology
Cornell University Medical College
Neurologist-in-Chief
The New York Hospital
New York, New York

PREFACE

During the course of our training, we frequently faced the lack of an easily accessible, succinct reference to the clinically relevant anatomic and physiologic details necessary for the immediate diagnosis and treatment of peripheral nerve disorders. Ideally, such a reference would bridge the gap between the Medical Research Council's concise *Aids to the Examination of the Peripheral Nervous System* and Haymaker and Woodhall's comprehensive *Peripheral Nerve Injuries*. This volume attempts such a synthesis, and also includes discussions of autonomic and reflex abnormalities. Our goal has been to construct a manual useful to students, house officers, and practitioners who care for patients with peripheral nerve disorders.

We owe our inspiration to the teachings of Drs. Fred Plum and Jerome Posner, who have instilled in all their students the physiologic and anatomic approach to clinical diagnosis and treatment of neurologic patients.

Edward Feldmann, M.D.
Orrin Devinsky, M.D.

CONTENTS

ANATOMY

CRANIAL NERVES AND SPINAL CORD

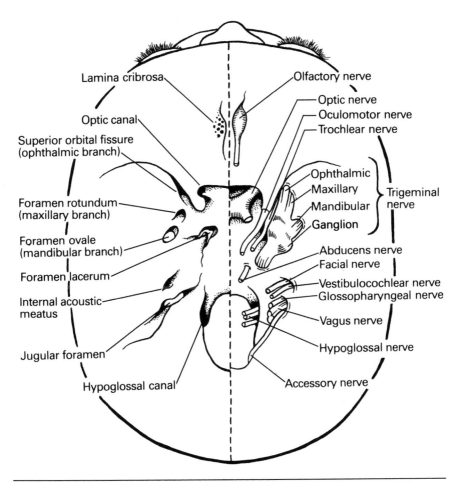

FIG. 1. Base of skull. On the left are shown the foramina of exiting and entering cranial nerves. On the right, the nerve stumps are shown. (Redrawn with modification from Duus P: Topical Diagnosis in Neurology. Georg Thieme Verlag, Stuttgart, 1983, p. 109.)

TABLE 1. The Cranial Nerves

CRANIAL NERVE	ORIGIN	FUNCTION	COURSE OF THE NERVE
I Olfactory (sensory)	Bipolar olfactory neurons	Smell	Central axons of bipolar neurons pass through cribriform plate of ethmoid bone and synapse in olfactory bulb
II Optic (sensory)	Retinal ganglion cells	Vision	Axons of ganglion cells converge at optic disc to form optic nerve, which passes through optic foramen
III Oculomotor Parasympathetic	Edinger-Westphal nucleus (upper midbrain)	Sphincter m. of iris, ciliary m.	Exits ventral midbrain near midline; runs parallel to posterior communicating artery, then traverses cavernous sinus & enters orbit through the superior orbital fissure
Motor	Oculomotor nucleus (upper midbrain)	Superior, inferior, and medial recti m.; inferior oblique m.; levator palpabrae superioris m.	
IV Trochlear (Motor)	Trochlear nucleus (lower midbrain)	Superior oblique m.	Fibers from the nucleus cross in anterior medullary velum and exit dorsally, below the colliculi; nerve traverses cavernous sinus after winding around midbrain; enters orbit through superior orbital fissure
V Trigeminal Motor	Motor nucleus of CN V (pons)	Muscles of mastication	
Sensory (somatic) see Fig. 1	Semilunar (trigeminal) ganglion	Tactile sensation to skin of face, mucosa of nose and mouth, and dura	Ophthalmic division (V1) passes through superior orbital fissure Maxillary division (V2) passes through foramen rotundum Mandibular division (V3) passes through foramen ovale
VI Abducens (Motor)	Abducens nucleus (pons)	Lateral rectus m.	Exits ventral pons near midline, ascends & curves around petrous tip; traverses cavernous sinus and enters orbit through superior orbital fissure. Long course
VII Facial Parasympathetic	Superior salivatory nucleus (pons)	Lacrimal gland & mucous membranes of mouth & nose; submandibular & sublingual salivary glands	Exits lower pons laterally and passes through internal auditory meatus into middle ear (where chorda tympani branch arises to carry taste fibers); then enters facial canal and exits cranium through stylomastoid foramen. Divides into terminal branches in the parotid gland
Motor	Main motor nucleus (pons)	Muscles of facial expression	
Sensory (somatic)	Geniculate ganglion	Tactile sensation to parts of external ear, auditory canal, & external tympanic membrane	

CN	Modality	Nucleus / Ganglion	Function	Notes
	Sensory (special)	Geniculate ganglion	Taste sensation to the anterior two-thirds of tongue	
VIII Vestibulocochlear	Vestibular n. (special sensory)	Vestibular ganglion	Equilibrium (supplies semicircular canals, utricle & saccule)	Vestibular and cochlear nerves join in the internal auditory meatus and enter the brain stem at the cerebellopontine angle
	Cochlear n. (special sensory)	Spiral ganglion	Hearing (supplies organ of Corti)	
IX Glossopharyngeal	Parasympathetic	Inferior salivatory nucleus (medulla)	Supplies parotid gland	Attaches to the rostral medulla near the posterolateral sulcus; exits cranium through jugular foramen
	Motor	Nucleus ambiguus (medulla)	Stylopharyngeus m.	
	Sensory (somatic)	Superior ganglion	Tactile sensation to posterior third of tongue, pharynx, middle ear, eustachian tube, & dura	
	Sensory (special)	Inferior ganglion	Taste sensation to the posterior third of tongue	
X Vagus	Parasympathetic	Dorsal motor nucleus of CN X (medulla)	Viscera of thorax & abdomen	Attaches to mid-medulla near the posterolateral sulcus; exits cranium through jugular foramen
	Motor	Nucleus ambiguus (medulla)	Muscles of pharynx & larynx	
	Sensory (somatic)	Superior ganglion	Tactile sensation to dura & auditory canal	
	Sensory (visceral afferents)	Inferior ganglion	Viscera of thorax & abdomen	
XI Accessory	Motor—cranial	Nucleus ambiguus (medulla)	Muscles of larynx	Cranial fibers pass in CN XI, then join CN X, and then in the recurrent laryngeal nerve. Spinal fibers ascend and enter cranium through the foramen magnum; then join the cranial fibers (in CN X) and exit the cranium through jugular foramen, and then separate from cranial fibers
	Motor—spinal	Anterior gray horn of cervical cord	Sternocleidomastoid & trapezius m.	
XII Hypoglossal (motor)		Hypoglossal nucleus (lower medulla)	Intrinsic muscles of tongue; genioglossus, hypoglossus, & styloglossus m.	Attaches to the lower medulla near the anterolateral sulcus; exits cranium through the hypoglossal canal (occipital bone)

n. = nerve; m. = muscle.

5

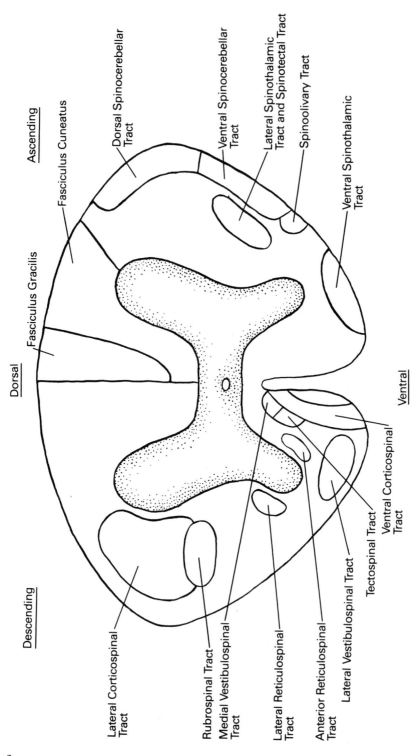

Ascending

Fasciculus Cuneatus

Dorsal Spinocerebellar Tract

Ventral Spinocerebellar Tract

Lateral Spinothalamic Tract and Spinotectal Tract

Spinoolivary Tract

Ventral Spinothalamic Tract

Fasciculus Gracilis

Dorsal

Ventral

Descending

Lateral Corticospinal Tract

Rubrospinal Tract
Medial Vestibulospinal Tract

Lateral Reticulospinal Tract

Anterior Reticulospinal Tract

Lateral Vestibulospinal Tract

Tectospinal Tract

Ventral Corticospinal Tract

FIG. 2. Cervical spinal cord. Descending tracts are shown on the left, ascending on the right.

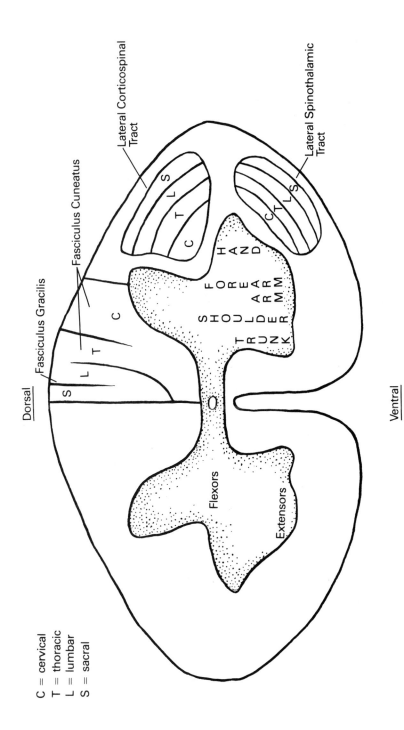

FIG. 3. Somatotopic organization of the cervical spinal cord. (Redrawn with modification from Romero-Sierra C: Neuroanatomy: A Conceptual Approach. Churchill Livingstone, New York, 1986, p. 87.)

C = cervical
T = thoracic
L = lumbar
S = sacral

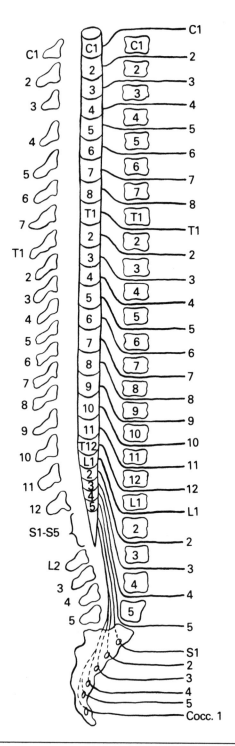

FIG. 4. The alignment of spinal segments and roots with vertebrae.

PLEXUSES

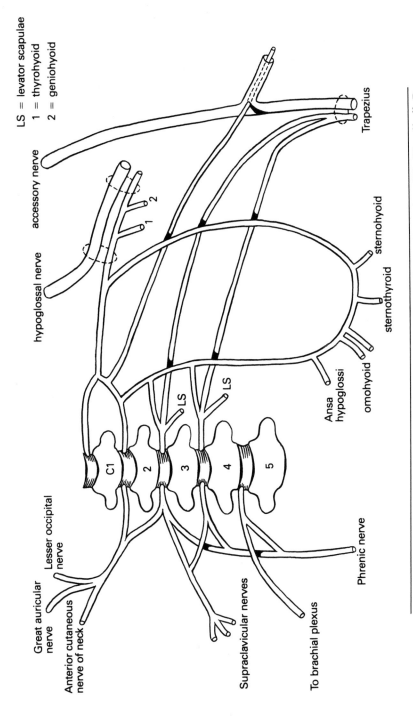

FIG. 5. The cervical plexus. (Redrawn with modification from Haymaker W, Woodhall B: Peripheral Nerve Injuries. WB Saunders, Philadelphia, 1953, p. 202.)

LS = levator scapulae
1 = thyrohyoid
2 = geniohyoid

accessory nerve

hypoglossal nerve

Trapezius

sternohyoid

sternothyroid

Ansa hypoglossi

omohyoid

LS

LS

C1

2

3

4

5

Great auricular nerve

Lesser occipital nerve

Anterior cutaneous nerve of neck

Supraclavicular nerves

Phrenic nerve

To brachial plexus

9

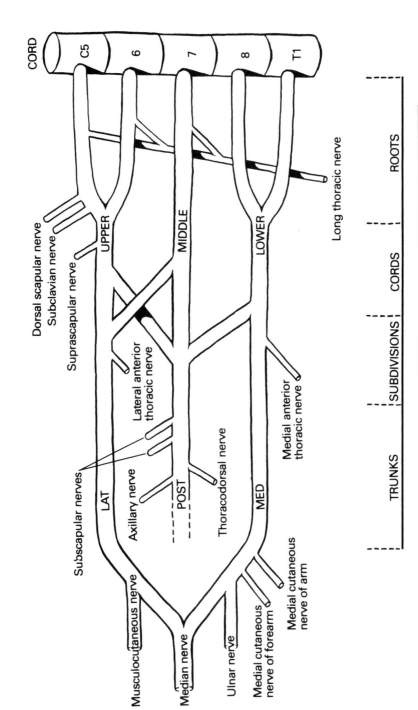

FIG. 6. The brachial plexus.

10

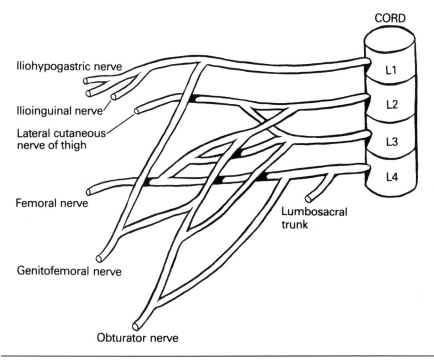

FIG. 7. The lumbar plexus.

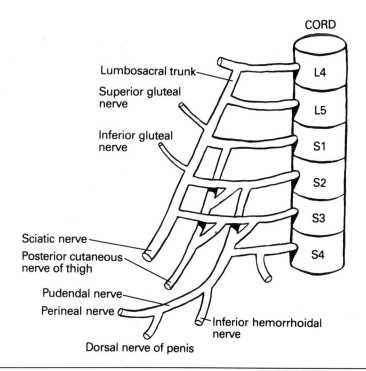

FIG. 8. The sacral plexus.

NERVES

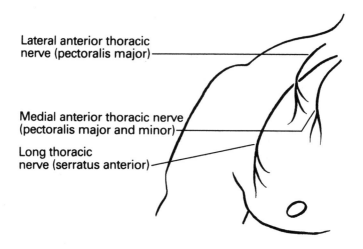

FIG. 9. Long thoracic (C5–7) and lateral and medial anterior thoracic (C5–T1) nerves.

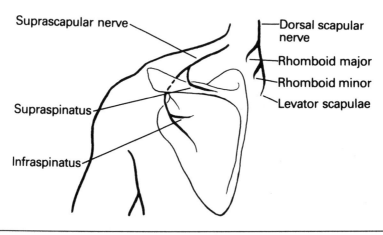

FIG. 10. Dorsal scapular (C3–6) and suprascapular (C5–6) nerves.

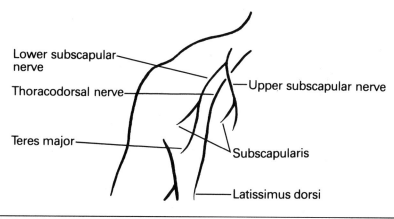

FIG. 11. Thoracodorsal (C6–8) and subscapular (C5–7) nerves.

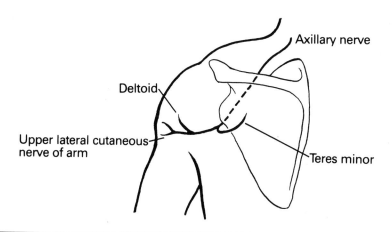

FIG. 12. Axillary nerve (C5–6).

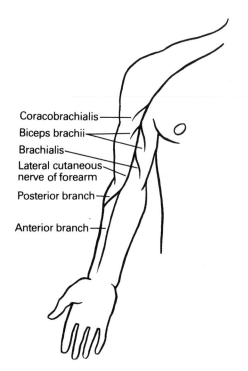

Coracobrachialis
Biceps brachii
Brachialis
Lateral cutaneous nerve of forearm
Posterior branch
Anterior branch

FIG. 13. Musculocutaneous nerve (C5–7).

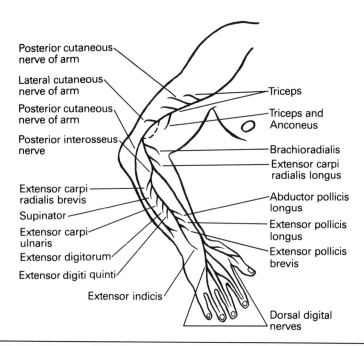

Posterior cutaneous nerve of arm
Lateral cutaneous nerve of arm
Posterior cutaneous nerve of arm
Posterior interosseus nerve
Extensor carpi radialis brevis
Supinator
Extensor carpi ulnaris
Extensor digitorum
Extensor digiti quinti
Extensor indicis

Triceps
Triceps and Anconeus
Brachioradialis
Extensor carpi radialis longus
Abductor pollicis longus
Extensor pollicis longus
Extensor pollicis brevis
Dorsal digital nerves

FIG. 14. Radial nerve (C5–8).

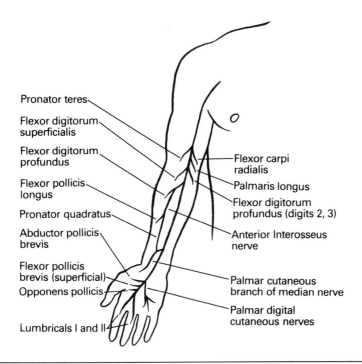

FIG. 15. Median nerve (C6–T1).

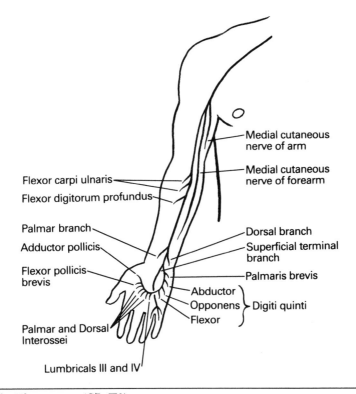

FIG. 16. Ulnar nerve (C7–T1).

15

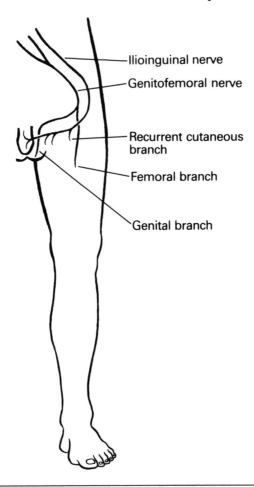

FIG. 17. Ilioinguinal (L1) and genitofemoral (L12) nerves.

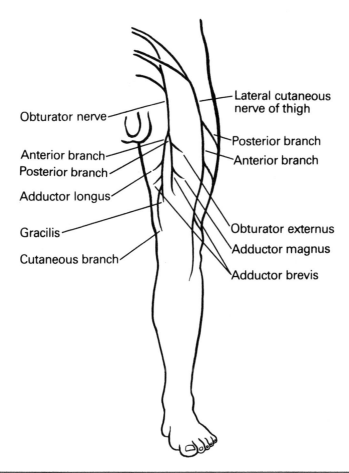

FIG. 18. Lateral femoral cutaneous nerve of thigh (L2–3) and obturator nerve (L2–4).

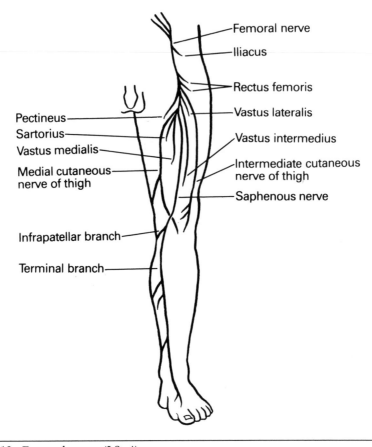

FIG. 19. Femoral nerve (L2–4).

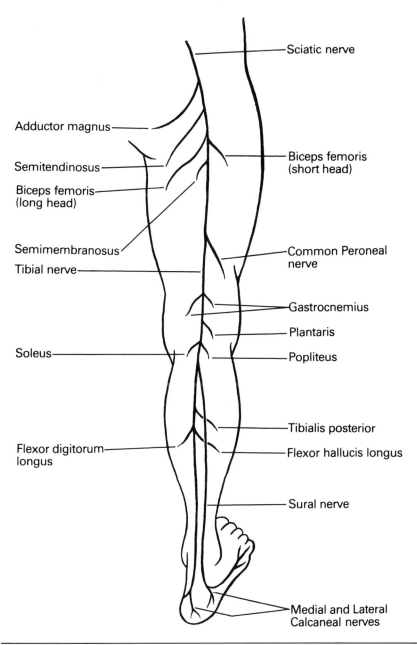

FIG. 20. Sciatic nerve (L4–S2).

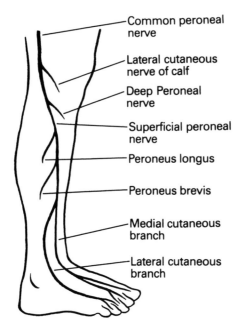

FIG. 21. Common peroneal and superficial peroneal nerves (L5–S1).

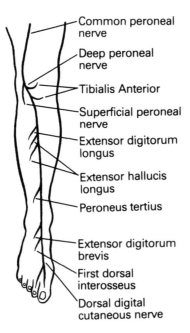

FIG. 22. Deep peroneal nerve (L4–S1).

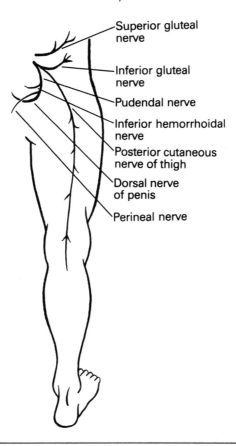

Superior gluteal
nerve

Inferior gluteal
nerve

Pudendal nerve

Inferior hemorrhoidal
nerve

Posterior cutaneous
nerve of thigh

Dorsal nerve
of penis

Perineal nerve

FIG. 23. Superior gluteal (L4–S1) and inferior gluteal (L5–S2) nerves.

SEGMENTAL AND PERIPHERAL INNERVATION OF MUSCLES

TABLE 2. Segmental and Peripheral Innervation of the Muscles and Their Function

NERVE/MUSCLE	FUNCTION	SPINAL SEGMENTS C3 C4 C5 C6 C7 C8 T1
Spinal accessory		
Trapezius	Elevates shoulder/arm Fixes scapula	C3 C4
Phrenic		
Diaphragm	Inspiration	C3 C4 C5
Dorsal scapular		
Rhomboids	Draw scapula up and in	C4 **C5** C6
Levator scapulae	Elevates scapula	C3 C4 C5
Long thoracic		
Serratus anterior	Fixes scapula on arm raise	C5 C6 C7
Anterior thoracic		
Pectoralis major (clavicular)	Pulls shoulder forward	**C5** C6
Pectoralis major (sternal)	Adducts and medially rotates arm	C6 **C7** C8 T1
Pectoralis minor	Depresses scapula, pulls shoulder forward	C6 C7 C8
Suprascapular		
Supraspinatus	Abducts humerus	**C5** C6
Infraspinatus	Rotates humerus laterally	**C5** C6
Subscapular		
Subscapularis	Rotates humerus medially	C5 C6
Teres major	Adducts, medially rotates humerus	C5 C6 C7
Thoracodorsal		
Latissimus dorsi	Adducts, medially rotates humerus	C6 **C7** C8
Axillary		
Teres minor	Adducts, laterally rotates humerus	C5 C6
Deltoid	Abducts arm	**C5** C6

22

Musculocutaneous		
Coracobrachialis	Flexes and adducts arm	C6**C7**
Biceps brachii	Flexes and supinates arm	C5C6
Brachialis	Flexes forearm	C5C6

Radial		
Triceps	Extends forearm	C6**C7**C8
Brachioradialis	Flexes forearm	C5**C6**
Extensor carpi radialis (longus and brevis)	Extend wrist, abduct hand	C5**C6**

Posterior interosseus		
Supinator	Supinates forearm	C6C7
Extensor carpi ulnaris	Extends wrist, adducts hand	**C7**C8
Extensor digitorum	Extends fingers at proximal phalanx	**C7**C8
Extensor digiti quinti	Extends little finger at proximal phalanx	**C7**C8
Abductor pollicis longus	Abducts thumb in the plane of palm	**C7**C8
Extensor pollicis (longus and brevis)	Extend thumb	**C7**C8
Extensor indicis	Extends index finger, proximal phalanx	**C7**C8

Median		
Pronator teres	Pronates and flexes forearm	C6C7
Flexor carpi radialis	Flexes wrist, abducts hand	C6C7
Palmaris longus	Flexes wrist	C7**C8**T1
Flexor digitorum superficialis	Flexes middle phalanges	C7**C8**T1
Flexor digitorum profundus (digits 2, 3)	Flexes distal phalanges	C7**C8**
Abductor pollicis brevis	Abducts thumb at right angles to palm	C8**T1**
Flexor pollicis brevis (superficial)	Flexes first phalanx of thumb	C8**T1**
Opponens pollicis	Flexes, opposes thumb	C8**T1**
Lumbricals (I,II)	Flex proximal interphalangeal joint, extend other phalanges	C8**T1**

Anterior interosseus		
Flexor digitorum profundus (digits 2,3)	Flexes distal phalanges	C7**C8**
Flexor pollicis longus	Flexes distal phalanx of thumb	C7**C8**
Pronator quadratus	Pronates forearm	C7**C8**T1

(Continues.)

Muscles are listed in the order of innervation, except when presented in groups as for the quadriceps. Boldface type signifies predominant innervation.

TABLE 2 (*Continued*). Segmental and Peripheral Innervation of the Muscles and Their Function

NERVE/MUSCLE	FUNCTION	SPINAL SEGMENTS C3C4C5C6C7C8T1
Ulnar		
Flexor carpi ulnaris	Flexes wrist, adducts hand	C7**C8**T1
Flexor digitorum profundus (digits 4,5)	Flexes distal phalanges	C7**C8**
Hypothenar muscles	Abduct, adduct, flex, rotate digit 5	C8**T1**
Lumbricals (III, IV)	Flex proximal interphalangeal joint, extend other phalanges	C8**T1**
Palmar interossei	Abduct fingers, flex proximal phalanges	C8**T1**
Dorsal interossei	Adduct fingers	C8**T1**
Flexor pollicis brevis (deep)	Flexes and adducts thumb	C8**T1**
Adductor pollicis	Adducts thumb	C8**T1**
		L1L2L3L4L5S1S2
Obturator		
Obturator externus	Adducts and outwardly rotates leg	**L2L3**L4
Adductor longus		
Adductor magnus	Adduct thigh	**L2L3**L4
Adductor brevis		
Gracilis		
Femoral		
Iliacus	Flexes leg at hip	L1**L2**L3
Rectus femoris		
Vastus lateralis	Extend leg	L2**L3L4**
Vastus intermedius		
Vastus medialis		
Pectineus	Adducts leg	**L2L3**L4
Sartorius	Inwardly rotates leg, flexes thigh and leg	**L2L3**L4
Sciatic		
Adductor magnus	Adducts thigh	L4L5S1
Semitendinosus	Flexes and medially rotates knee, extends hip	L5**S1**S2
Biceps femoris	Flexes leg, extends thigh	L5**S1**S2
Semimembranosus	Flexes and medially rotates knee, extends hip	L5**S1**S2

Nerve / Muscle	Action	Innervation
Tibial		
Gastrocnemius	Plantar flexes foot	S1S2
Plantaris	Spreads, brings together, and flexes proximal phalanges	L4L5S1
Soleus	Plantar flexes foot	S1S2
Popliteus	Plantar flexes foot	L4L5S1
Tibialis posterior	Plantar flexes and inverts foot	L4L5
Flexor digitorum longus	Flexes distal phalanges, aids plantar flexion	L5**S1S2**
Flexor hallucis longus	Flexes great toe, aids plantar flexion	L5**S1S2**
Small foot muscles	Cup sole	S1S2
Common peroneal		
Superficial peroneal		
Peroneus longus	Plantar flexes and everts foot	L5S1
Peroneus brevis	Plantar flexes and everts foot	L5S1
Deep peroneal		
Tibialis anterior	Dorsiflexes and inverts foot	**L4**L5
Extensor digitorum longus	Extends phalanges, dorsiflexes foot	**L5**S1
Extensor hallucis longus	Extends great toe, aids dorsiflexion	**L5**S1
Peroneus tertius	Plantar flexes foot in pronation	L4**L5**S1
Extensor digitorum brevis	Extends toes	L5S1
Superior gluteal		
Gluteus medius/minimus	Abduct and medially rotate thigh	**L4L5**S1
Tensor fasciae latae	Flexes thigh	**L4L5**S1
Inferior gluteal		
Gluteus maximus	Extends, abducts, laterally rotates thigh and extends lower trunk	**L5S1**S2

Muscles are listed in the order of innervation, except when presented in groups as for the quadriceps. Boldface type signifies predominant innervation.

TABLE 3. Segmental Innervation of Muscles

MUSCLE	SPINAL SEGMENTS C1 C2 C3 C4 C5 C6 C7 C8 T1
Sternocleidomastoid	C1 C2 C3 C4
Trapezius	C3 C4
Levator scapulae	C3 C4 C5
Diaphragm	C3 C4 C5
Rhomboids	C4 **C5** C6
Supraspinatus	**C5** C6
Infraspinatus	**C5** C6
Teres minor	C5 C6
Deltoid	**C5** C6
Biceps	C5 C6
Brachialis	C5 C6
Brachioradialis	C5 **C6**
Subscapularis	C5 C6
Extensor carpi radialis (longus and brevis)	C5 **C6**
Serratus anterior	C5 C6 C7
Teres major	C5 C6 C7
Pectoralis major	C5 C6 C7 C8 T1
Coracobrachialis	C6 **C7**
Supinator	C6 C7
Pronator teres	C6 C7
Flexor carpi radialis	C6 C7
Pectoralis minor	C6 C7 C8
Latissimus dorsi	C6 **C7** C8
Triceps	C6 **C7** C8
Extensor carpi ulnaris	**C7** C8
Extensor digitorum	**C7** C8
Extensor digiti quinti	**C7** C8
Abductor pollicis longus	**C7** C8
Extensor pollicis longus and brevis	**C7** C8
Extensor indicis	**C7** C8
Flexor digitorum profundus (all digits)	C7 **C8**
Flexor pollicis longus	C7 **C8**
Palmaris longus	C7 **C8** T1
Flexor digitorum superficialis	C7 **C8** T1
Pronator quadratus	C7 **C8** T1
Flexor carpi ulnaris	C7 **C8** T1
Abductor pollicis brevis	C8 **T1**
Flexor pollicis brevis (superficial and deep)	C8 **T1**
Opponens pollicis	C8 **T1**
Lumbricals (I–IV)	C8 **T1**
Hypothenar muscles	C8 **T1**
Palmar and dorsal interossei	C8 **T1**
Adductor pollicis	C8 **T1**

Boldface type signifies predominant innervation.   *(Continues.)*

TABLE 3 *(Continued).* Segmental Innervation of Muscles

MUSCLE	SPINAL SEGMENTS L1 L2 L3 L4 L5 S1 S2
Iliacus	**L1 L2**L3
Obturator externus	**L2 L3**L4
Adductor longus, brevis, magnus	**L2 L3**L4
Gracilis	**L2 L3**L4
Rectus femoris; vastus lateralis, intermedius, medialis	L2**L3 L4**
Pectineus	**L2 L3**L4
Sartorius	**L2 L3**L4
Tibialis posterior	L4 L5
Tibialis anterior	**L4**L5
Adductor magnus	L4 L5 S1
Plantaris	L4 L5 S1
Popliteus	L4 L5 S1
Peroneus tertius	L4 **L5**S1
Gluteus medius and minimus	**L4 L5**S1
Tensor fasciae latae	**L4 L5**S1
Peroneus longus and brevis	L5 S1
Extensor digitorum longus	**L5**S1
Extensor hallucis longus	**L5**S1
Extensor digitorum brevis	L5 S1
Semitendinosus	L5 **S1** S2
Biceps femoris	L5**S1**S2
Semimembranosus	L5**S1**S2
Flexor digitorum longus	L5**S1 S2**
Flexor hallucis longus	L5**S1 S2**
Gluteus maximus	**L5 S1**S2
Gastrocnemius	S1 S2
Soleus	S1 S2
Small foot muscles	S1 S2

TABLE 4. Muscles Acting on the Joints

Muscles Acting on the Temporomandibular Joint	Muscles Acting on the Shoulder Girdle and Joint

Open mouth
  Lateral pterygoids
  Digastric
  Geniohyoid
  Mylohyoid
	Elevation
	  Trapezius (upper fibers)
	  Sternocleidomastoid
	  Levator scapulae
	  Rhomboids—major and minor

Close mouth
  Masseter
  Temporalis
  Medial pterygoid
	Forward displacement (protraction)
	  Pectoralis minor
	  Serratus anterior

Protrude jaw
  Lateral pterygoids
  Medial pterygoids
	Backward displacement (retraction)
	  Trapezius
	  Rhomboids—major and minor

Laterally displace jaw toward opposite side
  Lateral pterygoid
  Medial pterygoid
	Flexion
	  Pectoralis major (clavicular fibers)
	  Coracobrachialis
	  Deltoid (anterior fibers)
	  Biceps

	Extension
	  Deltoid (posterior fibers)
	  Triceps
	  Teres major
	  Latissimus dorsi

	Adduction
	  Pectoralis major
	  Triceps
	  Teres major
	  Latissimus dorsi
	  Subscapularis

	Abduction
	  Deltoid
	  Supraspinatus

	Internal (medial) rotation
	  Pectoralis major
	  Deltoid (anterior fibers)
	  Teres major
	  Latissimus dorsi
	  Subscapularis

	External (lateral) rotation
	  Deltoid (posterior fibers)
	  Infraspinatus
	  Teres minor

Muscles Acting on the Elbow Joint

Extension
  Triceps
  Anconeus
  Extensor carpi radialis longus
  Extensor carpi radialis brevis
  Extensor carpi ulnaris
  Extensor digitorum
  Supinator

Flexion
  Biceps
  Brachialis
  Brachioradialis
  Flexor carpi radialis
  Flexor carpi ulnaris
  Pronator teres
  Flexor digitorum superficialis
  Palmaris longus

Supination
  Biceps
  Supinator
  Extensor pollicis longus

Pronation
  Pronator teres
  Pronator quadratus

Muscles Acting on the Wrist Joint

Flexion
  Flexor carpi ulnaris
  Flexor carpi radialis
  Palmaris longus
  Flexor digitorum profundus
  Flexor digitorum superficialis
  Flexor pollicis longus

Extension
  Extensor carpi ulnaris
  Extensor carpi radialis longus
  Extensor carpi radialis brevis
  Extensor digitorum
  Extensor pollicis longus
  Extensor indicis
  Extensor digiti minimi

Adduction
  Flexor carpi ulnaris
  Extensor carpi ulnaris

Abduction
  Extensor carpi radialis longus
  Extensor carpi radialis brevis
  Flexor carpi radialis
  Extensor pollicis longus
  Extensor pollicis brevis
  Abductor pollicis longus

Muscles Acting at the Finger Joints (Digits 2–5)

Flexion
  Flexor digitorum profundus (distal phalanges; digits 2–5)
  Flexor digitorum superficialis (middle and proximal phalanges, 2–5)
  Palmar interossei (proximal phalanges; digits 2, 4, 5)
  Dorsal interossei (proximal phalanges; digits 2–5)

Extension
  Extensor digitorum (all phalanges; digits 2–5)
  Extensor digiti minimi (all phalanges; digit 5)
  Extensor indicis (all phalanges; digit 2)
  Palmar interossei (distal phalanges; digits 2, 4, 5)
  Dorsal interossei (distal phalanges; digits 2–5)

Adduction
  Palmar interossei (digits 2, 4, 5)

Abduction
  Dorsal interossei (digits 2, 4, 5)
  Extensor digitorum (digits 2, 4, 5)
  Extensor digiti minimi (digit 5)
  Abductor digiti minimi (digit 5)
  Extensor indicis (digit 2)

Opposition
  Opponens digiti minimi (digit 5; draws metacarpal forward and rotates it medially)

(Continues.)

TABLE 4 *(Continued).* Muscles Acting on the Joints

Muscles Acting at the Thumb Joints	Muscles Acting on the Hip Joint

Muscles Acting at the Thumb Joints

Flexion
Flexor pollicis longus (both phalanges)
Flexor pollicis brevis (proximal phalanx
and metacarpal)
Opponens pollicis (metacarpal)

Extension
Extensor pollicis longus (both
phalanges and metacarpal)
Extensor pollicis brevis (proximal
phalanx and metacarpal)
Abductor pollicis longus (proximal
phalanx and metacarpal)

Adduction
Adductor pollicis (proximal phalanx)

Abduction
Abductor pollicis longus (metacarpal)
Abductor pollicis brevis (proximal
phalanx and metacarpal)

Opposition
Opponens pollicis (flexes metacarpal
and draws it medially)

Muscles Acting on the Hip Joint

Flexion
Iliacus
Rectus femoris
Pectineus
Sartorius
Tensor fasciae latae
Adductors

Extension
Gluteus maximus
Biceps femoris
Semimembranosus
Semitendinosus
Adductor magnus

Adduction
Adductor magnus
Adductor longus
Adductor brevis
Pectineus
Gracilis
Quadratus femoris
Obturator externus

Abduction
Gluteus medius
Gluteus minimus
Tensor fasciae latae
Piriformis
Sartorius

Medial (internal) rotation
Gluteus medius
Gluteus minimus
Tensor fasciae latae

Lateral (external) rotation
Obturator internus
Obturator externus
Piriformis
Gluteus maximus
Adductors
Gemelli
Quadratus femoris

Muscles Acting on the Knee Joint

Flexion
  Biceps femoris
  Semimembranosus
  Semitendinosus
  Gracilis
  Sartorius
  Gastrocnemius
  Popliteus
  Plantaris

Extension
  Quadricips femoris
  Tensor fasciae latae

Medial (internal) rotation
  Semimembranosus
  Semitendinosus
  Popliteus
  Gracilis
  Sartorius

Lateral (external) rotation
  Biceps femoris

Muscles Acting on the Ankle Joint

Dorsiflexion
  Tibialis anterior
  Extensor digitorum longus
  Extensor hallucis longus
  Peroneus tertius

Plantar flexion
  Soleus
  Gastrocnemius
  Tibialis posterior
  Flexor hallucis longus
  Plantaris
  Peroneus longus
  Peroneus brevis

Inversion
  Tibialis anterior
  Tibialis posterior
  Flexor digitorum (medial fibers)
  Flexor hallucis longus

Eversion
  Peroneus longus
  Peroneus brevis
  Extensor digitorum longus (lateral
    fibers)
  Peroneus tertius

Muscles Acting on the Toes

Flexion
  Flexor digitorum longus
  Flexor digitorum brevis
  Flexor hallucis longus
  Abductor hallucis
  Adductor hallucis
  Abductor digiti minimi
  Interossei (proximal phalanx)

Extension
  Extensor digitorum longus
  Extensor digitorum brevis
  Extensor hallucis longus
  Lumbricals
  Interossei (distal phalanges)

TABLE 5. Accessory Muscle Innervation

MUSCLE	NERVE	ACCESSORY SUPPLY
Platysma	Facial	C3–4
Trapezius, sternocleidomastoid	Accessory	C2–4
Diaphragm	Phrenic	Subclavian
Deltoid	Axillary	Anterior thoracic
Subscapularis	Subscapular	Axillary
Infraspinatus	Suprascapular	Axillary
Teres minor	Axillary	Suprascapular
Serratus anterior	Long thoracic	Dorsal scapular
Pectoralis major	Anterior thoracic	Axillary
Latissimus dorsi	Thoracodorsal	Axillary
Biceps	Musculocutaneous	Median
Brachialis	Musculocutaneous	Median
Triceps	Radial	Ulnar
Pronator teres	Median	Musculocutaneous
Flexor carpi radialis	Median	Musculocutaneous
Palmaris longus	Median	Musculocutaneous
Flexor digitorum digits 2 & 3	Median	Musculocutaneous
Flexor pollicis longus	Median	Musculocutaneous
Flexor pollicis brevis	Median	Ulnar
Opponens pollicis	Median	Ulnar
Abductor pollicis brevis	Median	Ulnar
Lumbricals I–II	Median	Ulnar
Flexor carpi ulnaris	Ulnar	Median
Flexor digitorum profundus, digits 4 & 5	Ulnar	Median
Adductor pollicis	Ulnar	Median
Lumbricals III–IV	Ulnar	Median
Interossei	Ulnar	Median
Adductor magnus	Obturator	Tibial

To diagnose which nerve is injured requires knowledge of the exact muscular innervation. However, there is a variability in the innervation of motor fibers as certain muscles may receive accessory innervation. The most common accessory innervations of specific muscles are presented in this table.

SENSORY INNERVATION OF THE HEAD AND NECK

IO = infraorbital
IT = infratrochlear
L = lacrimal
NC = nasociliary
ST = supratrochlear
ZF = zygomaticofacial
ZT = zygomaticotemporal

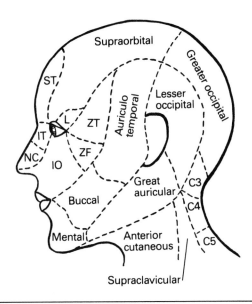

FIG. 24. Cutaneous innervation of the head and neck. (Redrawn with modification from Haymaker W, Woodhall B: Peripheral Nerve Injuries. WB Saunders, Philadelphia, 1953, p. 39.)

I = ophthalmic
II = maxillary
III = mandibular

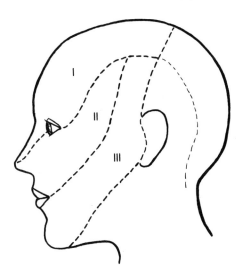

FIG. 25. Cutaneous fields of the head supplied by the three divisions of the trigeminal nerve.

DERMATOMES

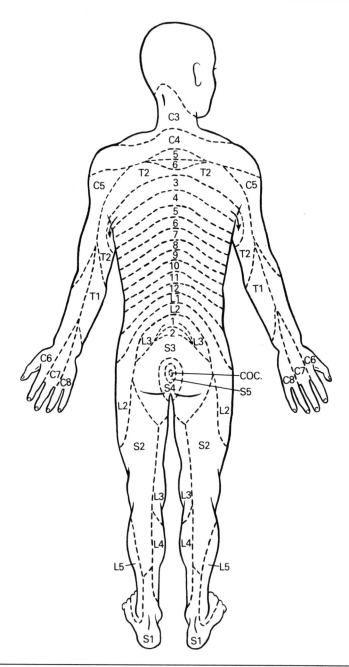

FIG. 26. The dermatomes from the back. (Redrawn with modification from Haymaker W, Woodhall B: Peripheral Nerve Injuries. WB Saunders, Philadelphia, 1953, p. 26.)

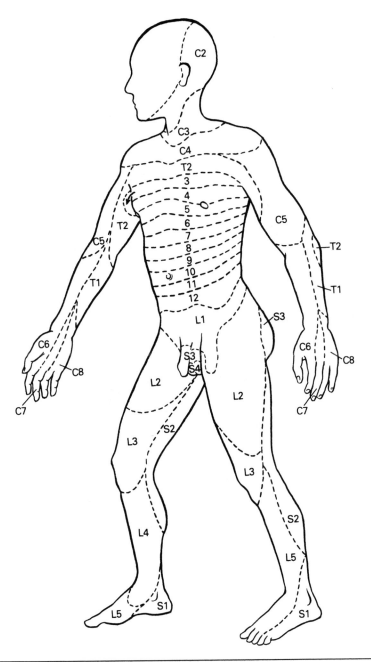

FIG. 27. A side view of the dermatomes. (Redrawn with modification from Haymaker W, Woodhall B: Peripheral Nerve Injuries. WB Saunders, Philadelphia, 1953, p. 27.)

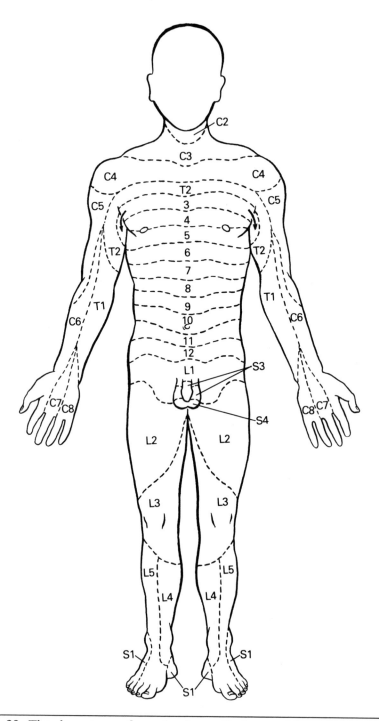

FIG. 28. The dermatomes from the front. (Redrawn with modification from Haymaker W, Woodhall B: Peripheral Nerve Injuries. WB Saunders, Philadelphia, 1953, p. 28.)

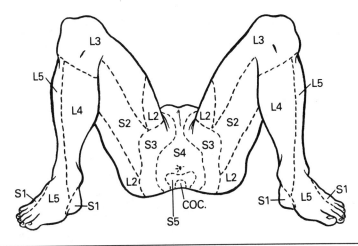

FIG. 29. The dermatomes of the perineum and limbs. (Redrawn with modification from Haymaker W, Woodhall B: Peripheral Nerve Injuries. WB Saunders, Philadelphia, 1953, p. 29.)

SENSORY FIELDS OF PERIPHERAL NERVES

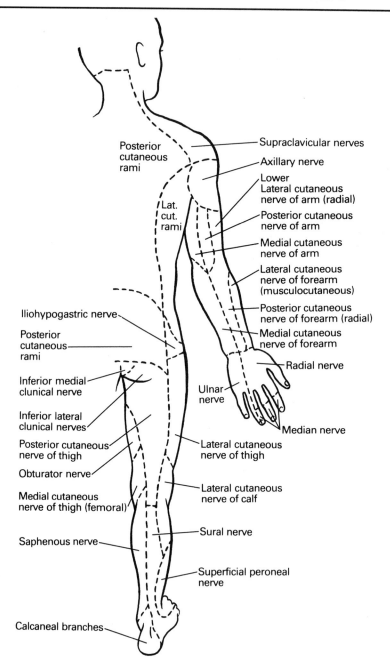

FIG. 30. The cutaneous fields of the peripheral nerves from the back. (Redrawn with modification from Haymaker W, Woodhall B: Peripheral Nerve Injuries. WB Saunders, Philadelphia, 1953, p. 40.)

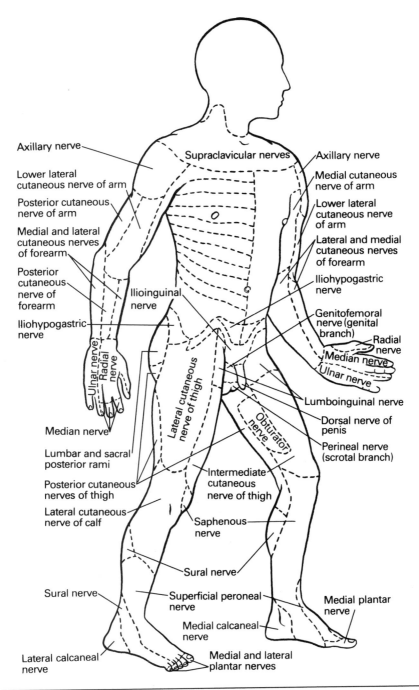

FIG. 31. Side view of the cutaneous fields of the peripheral nerves. The fields of the intercostal nerves are indicated by numerals. (Redrawn with modification from Haymaker W, Woodhall B: Peripheral Nerve Injuries. WB Saunders, Philadelphia, 1953, p. 42.)

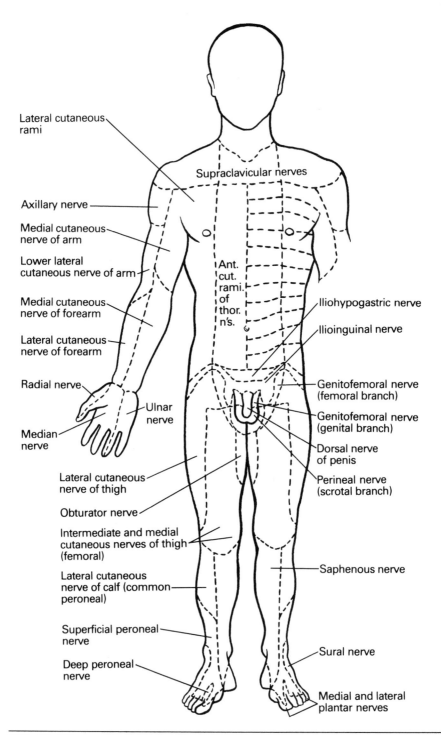

FIG. 32. The cutaneous field of peripheral nerves from the front. (Redrawn with modification from Haymaker W, Woodhall B: Peripheral Nerve Injuries. WB Saunders, Philadelphia, 1953, p. 43.)

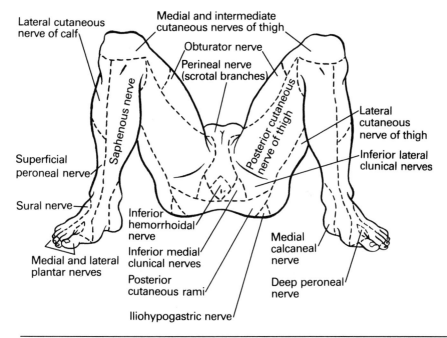

FIG. 33. Peripheral nerve fields of the perineum and limbs. (Redrawn with modification from Haymaker W, Woodhall B: Peripheral Nerve Injuries. WB Saunders, Philadelphia, 1953, p. 44.)

AUTONOMOUS ZONES

The anatomic fields supplied by adjacent cutaneous nerves overlap to a considerable extent and, therefore, the region of sensory loss following nerve section is smaller than the cutaneous area supplied by the nerve. The area of complete sensory loss corresponds to the area supplied exclusively by the interrupted nerve and is called the *autonomous zone*. Remember, in most injuries the area of pinprick loss is smaller than the area of tactile and thermal anesthesia.

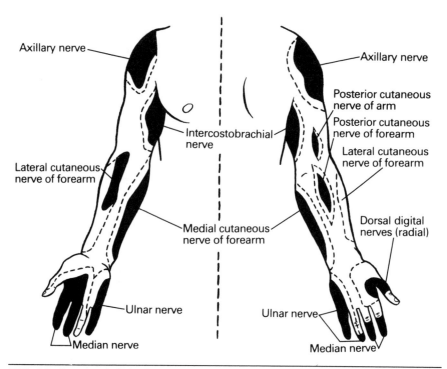

FIG. 34. Sensory deficit after interruption of individual nerve trunks of the upper limb. The black areas represent the autonomous zones and the surrounding dotted lines show the approximate border of tactile anesthesia and thermoanesthesia. (Redrawn with modification from Haymaker W, Woodhall B: Peripheral nerve Injuries. WB Saunders, Philadelphia, 1953, p. 138.)

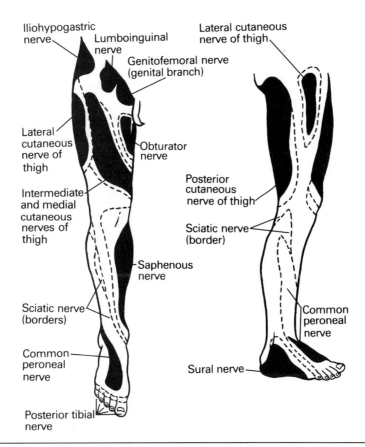

FIG. 35. Sensory deficit following interruption of individual nerve trunks of the lower limb. (Redrawn with modification from Haymaker W, Woodhall B: Peripheral Nerve Injuries. WB Saunders, Philadelphia, 1953, p. 140.)

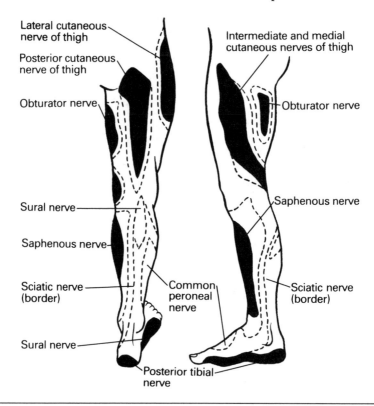

FIG. 36. Sensory deficit following interruption of individual nerve trunks of the lower limb. (Redrawn with modification from Haymaker W, Woodhall B: Peripheral Nerve Injuries. WB Saunders, Philadelphia, 1953, p. 141.)

TABLE 6. Typical Clinical Deficits Seen with Proximal Nerve Lesions

NERVE	IMPAIRMENT
Musculocutaneous	Forearm flexion at elbow, supination
Radial	Forearm extension, flexion, supination Wrist extension Thumb extension, abduction in plane of palm
Median	Forearm pronation Wrist flexion Finger flexion (digits 2, 3) Thumb flexion, opposition, abduction at right angle to palm
Ulnar	Wrist flexion, adduction Abduction and adduction of all digits Finger flexion (digits 4, 5) Flex, rotate digit 5
Obturator	Thigh adduction
Femoral	Thigh flexion at hip Leg extension at knee
Sciatic	Leg flexion at knee
Tibial	Foot plantar flexion, inversion Toe flexion, cup sole
Superficial peroneal	Foot eversion
Deep peroneal	Foot dorsiflexion, toe extension

SCLEROTOMES AND PERIPHERAL BONE INNERVATION

Sclerotomes are areas of segmental innervation of bone. Traumatic lesions of bones, tendons, ligaments, and fasciae may produce pain that is referred to the sclerotomes. Usually no sensorimotor or reflex changes occur. The peripheral nerve innervation of the skeleton closely follows muscle innervation; that is, the bones are innervated by the same nerves that supply the muscles attached to that bone. Injury of peripheral nerves may lead to osteoporosis, fibrosis, or ankylosis of the innervated bones, joints, and periarticular tissues.

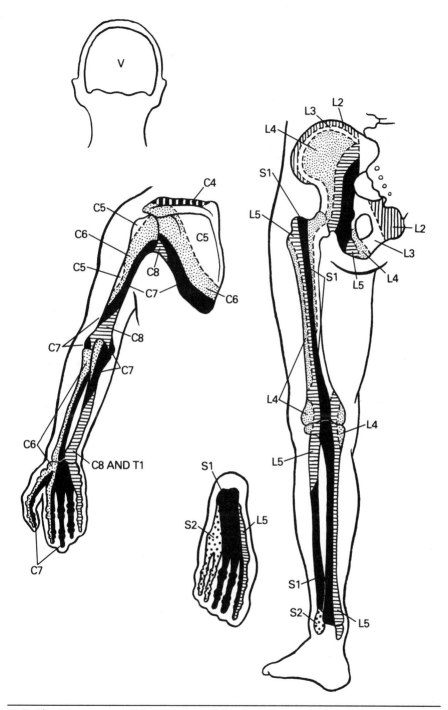

FIG. 37. The segmental innervation of the skeleton, posterior view. The patterns indicate the segmental supply. The skull is innervated by the trigeminal. The vertebrae are supplied by posterior primary rami of the respective spinal nerves, the ribs by both posterior and anterior primary rami. (Redrawn with modification from Haymaker W, Woodhall B: Peripheral Nerve Injuries. WB Saunders, Philadelphia, 1953, p. 48.)

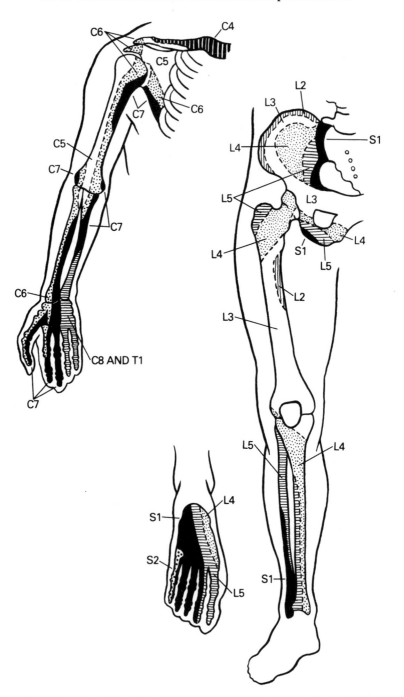

FIG. 38. Segmental skeletal innervation, anterior view. The sclerotomes are indicated by the various styles of shading. (Redrawn with modification from Haymaker W, Woodhall B: Peripheral Nerve Injuries. WB Saunders, Philadelphia, 1953, p. 49.)

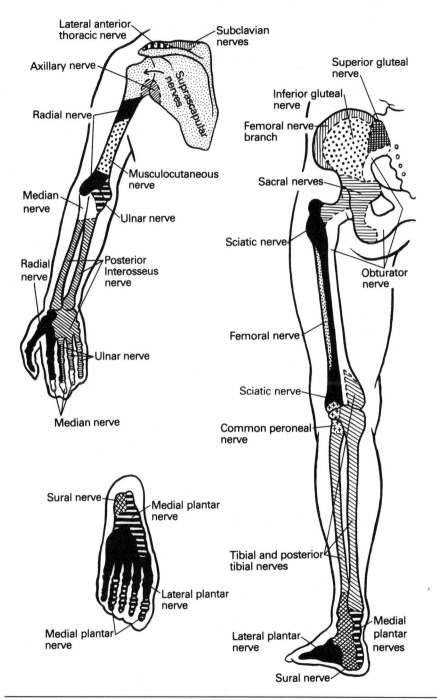

FIG. 39. The peripheral nerve supply of the skeleton, posterior view. (Redrawn with modification from Haymaker W, Woodhall B: Peripheral Nerve Injuries. WB Saunders, Philadelphia, 1953, p. 50.)

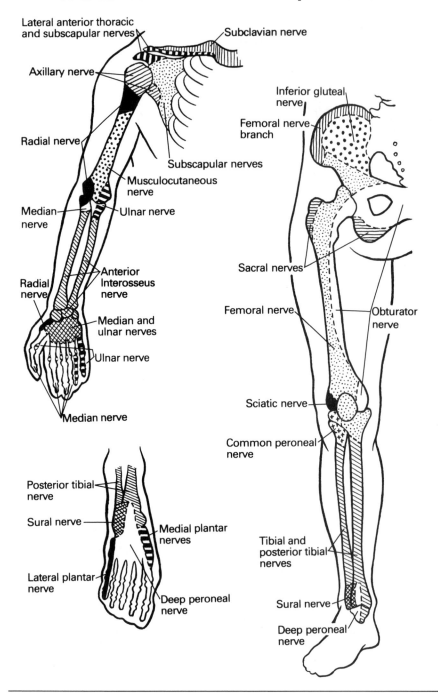

FIG. 40. The peripheral nerve supply of the skeleton, anterior view. (Redrawn with modification from Haymaker W, Woodhall B: Peripheral Nerve Injuries. WB Saunders, Philadelphia, 1953, p. 51.)

PATTERNS
FOR REFERRED PAIN

Visceral afferents for pain may be "felt" or "referred" to somatic areas that have a similar representation in the spinal cord. Typically the pain is felt in a small area of skin or myofascial tissue that is supplied by the same or adjacent spinal segment. Common patterns include

Diaphragm	C4
Heart	C8–T8 (chest, left arm, jaw, epigastrium)
Stomach	T6–9
Intestine	T7–10
Rectum	S2–4
Bladder	T2–10
Prostate/testes/uterus	T10–12
Kidneys	T11–L1

TABLE 7. The Superficial Cutaneous Reflexes

REFLEX	EXAMINATION	EFFECT	LOCALIZATION
Corneal	Touch corneoscleral junction	Bilateral eyelid closure	CNs V and VII
Palatal/pharyngeal	Touch soft palate and pharynx	Palate elevation and gagging	CNs IX and X
Palmar	Stroke palmar surface of hand	Finger flexion	C8–T1
Abdominal	Stroke skin of abdomen: upper	Abdominal wall contraction	Upper T7–9
	middle		Middle T9–11
	lower		Lower T11–L1
Cremasteric	Stroke medial upper thigh	Scrotal and testicular elevation	L1–2
Gluteal	Stroke skin of buttocks	Gluteal contraction	L4–S1
Plantar	Stroke sole of foot	Toe flexion	S1–2
Babinski[a]	Stroke sole of foot	Dorsiflexion of great toe, fanning of other toes, dorsiflexion of ankle, flexion of knee and hip	Pyramidal tract lesion above L4
Chaddock[a]	Stroke lateral aspect of foot		
Oppenheim[a]	Run hand down over anterior tibia		
Gordon[a]	Squeeze calf muscles		
Bulbocavernosus	Pressure on glans penis	Contraction of bulbocavernosus	S3–4
Anal	Stroke perianal region	Contraction of external anal sphincter	S2–4

[a] Reflexes not present in normal individuals.

TABLE 8. The Muscle Stretch Reflexes

REFLEX	EXAMINATION	EFFECT	LOCALIZATION
Jaw jerk	Tap center of slightly opened lower jaw	Jaw closure	CN V
Orbicularis oculi	Fold skin over temple between fingers; strike fingers	Contraction of both orbicularis oculi muscles	CN VII
Head retraction[a]	Tap maxilla beneath nose with head slightly bent	Involuntary backward head jerk	Bilateral supracervical pyramidal tract
Sternocleidomastoid	Tap muscle at clavicular origin	Muscle contraction	C3–4
Pectoral	Arm abducted, tap finger over tendon to humerus	Adduction, internal rotation of arm	C5–T1
Biceps	Tap thumb placed over biceps tendon	Elbow flexion	C5–6
Brachioradialis	With forearm semipronated, tap styloid process of radius	Elbow flexion	C5–6
Scapulohumeral	Tap medial, lower scapula	Adduction or abduction of arm	C5–7
Pronator	Tap palmar forearm medial to styloid process of radius	Forearm pronation	C6
Triceps	Tap just above olecranon	Elbow extension	C6–7
Finger flexion	Tap ends of semiflexed fingers	Finger flexion	C6–T1
Abdominal muscle	Tap ruler pressed on abdomen, costal margin in nipple line, or symphysis pubis	Abdominal wall contraction	T7–L1
Adductor	Tap medial condyle of femur	Leg adduction	L2–4
Patellar	Tap patellar tendon	Knee extension	L2–4
Tibialis posterior	Tap above and behind medial malleolus	Foot inversion	L5–S1
Biceps femoris	Tap head of fibula	Posterior upper leg contraction	L5–S2
Achilles (triceps surae)	Tap Achilles tendon	Foot plantar flexion	S1–2

[a] Reflex not seen in normal individuals.

AUTONOMIC NERVOUS SYSTEM

TABLE 9. Autonomic Nervous System—Physiology and Anatomy

TISSUE SUPPLIED	PARASYMPATHETIC NERVOUS SYSTEM			SYMPATHETIC NERVOUS SYSTEM		
	STIMULATION	PREGANGLIONIC NEURON	POSTGANGLIONIC NEURON	STIMULATION[a]	PREGANGLIONIC NEURON[b]	POSTGANGLIONIC NEURON
Eye						
Ciliary m.	Contraction (near vision)	Edinger-Westphal n. (midbrain)	Ciliary ganglion	Relaxation (β)	IMLN C8–T2[b]	Superior cervical ganglion
Constrictor m. of iris	Contraction (miosis)	Edinger-Westphal n. (midbrain)	Ciliary ganglion	—	—	—
Dilator (radial) m. of iris	—	—	—	Contraction (α)	IMLN C8–T2	Superior cervical ganglion
Lacrimal gland	Secretion	Superior salivatory n. (pons); CN VII	Pterygopalatine ganglion	—	—	—
Salivary glands						
Parotid	Secretion	Inferior salivatory n. (medulla); CN IX	Otic ganglion	Secretion (α & β)	IMLN T1–3	Superior & middle cervical ganglia
Submandibular & sublingual	Secretion	Superior salivatory n. (pons); CN VII	Submandibular ganglion	Secretion (α & β)	IMLN T1–3	Superior & middle cervical ganglia
Sweat glands						
Head & neck	—	—	—	Secretion	IMLN T1–3	All cervical ganglia Paravertebral ganglia
Body & limbs	Slight secretion	—	—	Secretion	IMLN C8–L2	
Bronchial muscle	Contraction	Dorsal motor n. of CN X (medulla)	Pulmonary plexi	Relaxation (β_2)	IMLN T1–5	Inferior cervical & paravertebral ganglia
Heart	Decreased heart rate, AV node conduction time, & contractility	Dorsal motor n. of CN X (medulla)	Cardiac ganglia (mainly atrial)	Increased heart rate, contractility, automaticity, & conduction	IMLN T1–6	All cervical & paravertebral ganglia

	Parasympathetic action	Parasympathetic origin	Parasympathetic ganglia	Sympathetic action	Sympathetic origin	Sympathetic ganglia
Arterioles						
Viscera & skeletal muscle	—	—	—	Constriction (α) Dilation (β_2)	IMLN C8–L2	Paravertebral ganglia
Cerebral & skin	—	—	—	Constriction (α)	IMLN C8–L2	Paravertebral ganglia
Veins	—	—	—	Constriction (α) Dilation (β_2)	IMLN C8–L2	Paravertebral ganglia
GI tract						
Esophagus through transverse colon	Increase in tone & motility; decrease in sphincter tone	Dorsal motor n. of CN X (medulla)	Local GI ganglia	Decrease tone & motility (α_2, β_2); increase sphincter tone (α_1)	IMLN T1–11	Thoracic paravertebral, celiac, and superior mesenteric ganglia
Descending colon & rectum	Increase in tone & motility; decrease in sphincter tone	Intermediate gray S2–4	Local GI ganglia	Decrease tone & motility (α_2, β_2); increase sphincter tone (α_1)	IMLN T12–L2	Lumbar paravertebral & inferior mesenteric ganglia
Bladder						
Detrusor muscle	Contraction	Intermediate gray S2–4 (pelvic nerve)	Ganglia in bladder wall	Minimal relaxation (β_2)	IMLN T12–L2	Lumbar paravertebral & inferior mesenteric ganglia
Internal sphincter	Relaxation	Intermediate gray S2–4 (pelvic nerve)	Ganglia in bladder wall	Contraction (α)	IMLN T12–L2	Lumbar paravertebral & inferior mesenteric ganglia
Genitalia	Erection	Intermediate gray S2–4 (pelvic nerve)	Local ganglia	Ejaculation (α)	IMLN T12–L2	Lumbar paravertebral & inferior mesenteric ganglia

[a] α = adrenergic; β = adrenergic.
[b] IMLN = intermediolateral nucleus.
m. = muscle; n. = nerve.

EXAMINATION

GENERAL PRINCIPLES
OF EXAMINATION

I. *History.* A careful history is an essential prerequisite to the examination. Specifically, weakness, fatigue, adventitious movements, cramping, pain, sensory loss, and spontaneous sensations (hallucinations) or distortions (illusions) should be elicited. If there is a positive response, explore the associated features—first episode, precipitants, mode of onset, duration, etc. If sensory loss is reported ask the patient to map its distribution; after your examination leave the patient a pin and cotton-tip swab with which to carefully remap the region.

While taking the history, form hypotheses regarding the pathophysiology of the symptoms. Consider nonneurologic syndromes (e.g., claudication causing fatigable lower extremity "weakness," fatigability in depression or lupus misrepresented as focal weakness). In the differential diagnosis of neurologic causes, first localize the level of the lesion. Be systematic. Start at the muscle and work centrally—i.e., muscle—neuromuscular junction—peripheral nerve—plexus—root—cord—brain stem—diencephalon—cerebrum. The most common errors are (1) locating the lesion in the central nervous system when it is actually peripheral, (2) making an etiologic diagnosis before localizing the lesion, and (3) once reaching a "diagnosis," accepting it de facto; failing to pause, play devil's advocate, and consider that you may be wrong.

II. Before beginning the examination, make sure the patient is comfortable. A motor or sensory examination performed on an exhausted or acutely ill patient yields limited and often misleading information. Such patients can be briefly screened and then reexamined when conditions are more favorable. Similarly, the examiner should not be exhausted, hurried or distracted (a condition hard to achieve in the age of the *beeper*). When a detailed examination is required it may be wise to give the patient and examiner a rest in the middle and complete the exam later.

III. The examination

    A. *Observe carefully—both before and during tests of tone and muscle strength.* The patient must disrobe so that the area of interest is fully exposed and the two sides can be compared.

        1. *Skin.* Check color, moistness (tested by touch or by comparing the ease with which the drum of the vibrating fork can be slid across the skin), texture; check for stigmata of minor trauma (often associated with deafferentation).

        2. *Muscle bulk.* Compare the two sides to each other and to the norm given the patient's age, sex, nutritional status, and level of physical activity.

3. *Resting posture.* Check the patient's resting posture (for example, flexion of the arm/wrist/fingers and external rotation of the lower extremity in the supine position suggested corticospinal lesions); check for splinting with pain, dystonia.
4. *Spontaneous movements.* Are they fluid? Is there hesitation? Are they pain limited? Is the patient hypo- or hyperkinetic?
5. *Adventitious movement.* Note tremor, fasciculation, fibrillation, tic, dyskinesia, myokymia, cramps, myoclonus, spasms, athetosis, chorea.

B. Palpate

1. For tone
2. For nerves:

   a. *Ulnar nerve.* Palpate the ulnar nerve in the condylar (ulnar) groove, between the medial epicondyle of the humerus and the insertion of the triceps on the olecranon.
   b. *Peroneal nerve.* Locate the peroneal nerve in the fibular tunnel, as the nerve winds laterally around the neck of the fibula (passing through the origin of the superficial head of the peroneus longus).

IV. The motor examination

A. The motor examination has three parts—observation, palpation, and testing for myotonia and strength

B. *Myotonia.* Myotonia is an increase in muscle irritability and contractility evident on active rather than passive movement; it is associated with decreased power of muscle relaxation (the handshake that won't let go!).

1. *Percussion myotonia.* Percussion myotonia is elicited by mechanical stimulation. Using the reflex hammer, deliver an abrupt tap. If percussion myotonia is present, the tap will produce an indentation or dimpling that gradually disappears; tapping on the thenar eminence may cause thumb opposition lasting seconds.
2. Myotonia is present in congenital and acquired forms of myotonia, myotonic dystrophy, and paramyotonia, and in some cases of myxedema.

C. Muscle strength

1. *Grading.* The British system most commonly used:
   0   No contraction
   1   Flicker/trace of contraction
   2   Active movement with gravity eliminated

3 Active movement against gravity

4 Active movement against gravity and resistance

5 Normal power

Note. Grade 4 is often subdivided into 4 − (slight), 4 (moderate), and 4 + (good) resistance; grade 5 − is used to denote minimal decrease in power, often reflecting an asymmetry or the ability to "break" a muscle with great effort in a very strong person.

2. Tips for muscle testing

    a. Test muscles in the order in which motor branches enter them from the parent nerve (for example, when testing radial nerve innervation, check muscles in the order triceps, brachioradialis, extensor carpi radialis, etc.).

    b. Eliminate gravity, put muscle at no advantage.

    c. Test strength at a specific point; remember that work is equal to force times distance. Thus, a frail examiner can "break" the abducted arm of a weight lifter by pushing down on the hand (a distal point), whereas even a muscle-bound examiner may have difficulty "breaking" the abducted arm of a frail patient by pushing down on the uppermost arm. Try to be consistent in your technique.

    d. Is pain limiting muscular effort?

    e. Is a limited range of motion affecting performance?

    f. Are trick movements—performed by synergist muscles—being mistaken for actions of the prime mover?

    g. Is the weakness functional (hysteria or malingering)? Use specific maneuvers to check. In functional weakness there is often simultaneous contraction of agonists and antagonists; thus, after suddenly removing support from a limb (e.g., an arm abducted 90 degrees) it will briefly hold its position. The patient may be unable to make specific movements (e.g., wrist extension) but use these muscles as synergists (e.g., in making a fist). *The diagnosis of functional disease should be made with extreme caution.*

    h. Is tendon or ligament injury presenting as "nerve palsy"?

    i. Consider nerve injury associated with fracture, splint, and vascular injury.

    j. Is contracture secondary to scar, vascular injury, or ankylosis, rather than being caused by a primary nerve injury?

    k. Arthropathy and deformities after peripheral nerve injury should be considered.

MOTOR TESTING BY MUSCLE/MOVEMENT

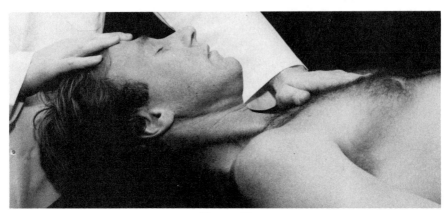

Figure 41

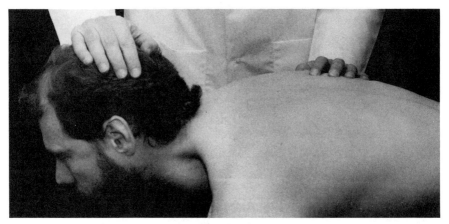

Figure 42

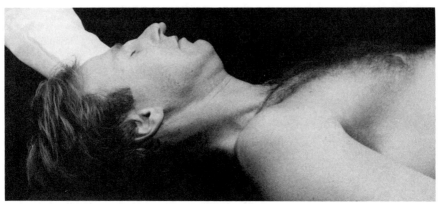

Figure 43

FIG. 41 Neck flexion

Sternocleidomastoid (CN XI and C2–4)*
Scaleni muscles (C3–8)

The patient flexes the head forward against resistance (ask the patient to move chin towards the chest). Deviation of the head toward one side results from weakness of the ipsilateral sternocleidomastoid.

FIG. 42 Neck extension

Trapezius (CN XI and C3–4)
Splenius capitis (C2–4)
Splenius cervicis (C3–6)
Intertransversarii (C2–8)
Upper part of sacrospinalis (erector spinae; C2–8)

The patient moves the head backward against resistance (ask the patient to move occiput towards back).

FIG. 43 Lateral rotation of the neck

Sternocleidomastoid (CN XI and C2–4)
Scaleni muscles (C3–8)

The examiner places his hand on the patient's lower face and asks the patient to rotate the head toward that side.

---

* Muscles printed in boldface are the primary muscles responsible for the action.

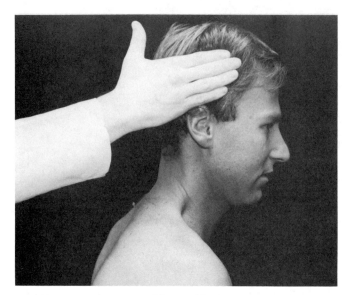

Figure 44

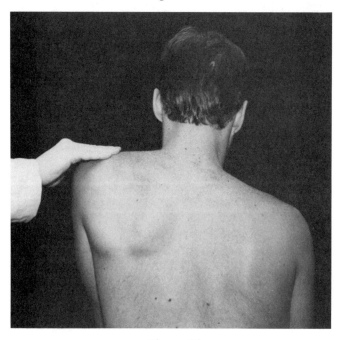

Figure 45

FIG. 44 Lateral flexion (abduction) of the neck

Sternocleidomastoid (CN XI and C2–4)
Scaleni muscles (C3–8)

The examiner places his hand above the ear and resists as the patient tries to bring the ear towards the shoulder.

FIG. 45 Shoulder elevation (shrug)

Upper half of trapezius (CN XI and C3–4)
Levator scapulae (C3–5)

The patient shrugs (elevates) the shoulder against resistance.

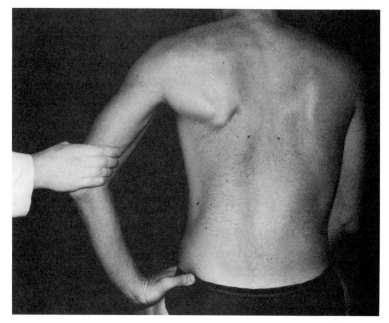

Figure 46

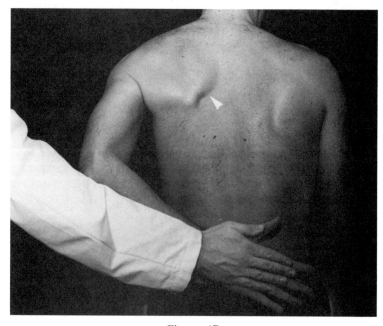

Figure 47

FIG. 46 Bracing of the shoulder (retraction/abduction of scapula)

Rhomboids (dorsal scapular nerve, C4–6)
Lower two-thirds of trapezius (CN XI and C3–4)
Latissimus dorsi (thoracodorsal nerve, C6–8)

The patient attempts to move the shoulder backward against resistance.

FIG. 47 Rhomboids test

Rhomboids (dorsal scapular nerve, C4–6)

The patient places his hand behind the back and the palm is then pushed backward against resistance.

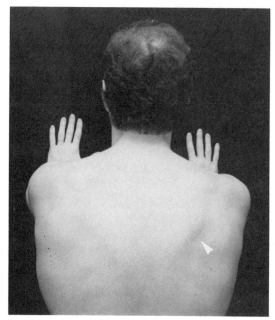

Figure 48

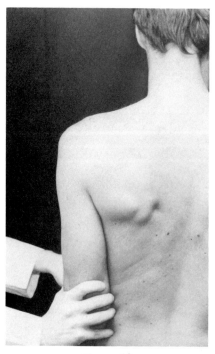

Figure 49

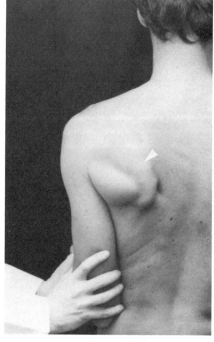

Figure 50

FIG. 48 The pushing test

Serratus anterior (long thoracic nerve, C5–7)

The patient pushes the palms of the extended arm against a wall. Normally the medial border of the scapula remains close to the chest wall and the lower fibers of the trapezius can be seen and palpated (arrow). With weakness of the serratus anterior, the inferior angle of the scapula deviates medially and the superomedial border deviates laterally ("winging").

FIG. 49 Medial (internal) rotation of the arm at the shoulder.

Subscapularis (subscapular nerves, C5–6)
Teres major (lower subscapular nerve, C5–7)
Anterior fibers of deltoid (axillary nerve, C5–6)
Latissimus dorsi (thoracodorsal nerve, C6–8)
Pectoralis major (lateral and medial anterior thoracic nerves, C5–T1)

The patient supinates and flexes the forearm at a right angle and medially rotates the arm at the shoulder against resistance. Note: in the upright position, gravity will facilitate this movement. If weakness is detected, each muscle should be palpated to determine which are involved.

FIG. 50 Lateral (external) rotation of the arm at the shoulder

Infraspinatus (suprascapular nerve, C5–6)
Teres minor (axillary nerve, C5–6)
Posterior fibers of deltoid (axillary nerve, C5–6)

The patient supinates and flexes the forearm at a right angle and laterally rotates the arm at the shoulder against resistance. The examiner should stand behind the patient to see and palpate the contraction of the infraspinatus.

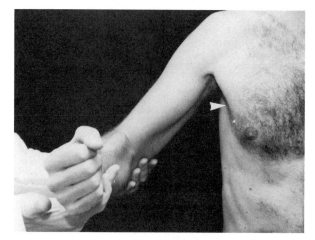

Figure 51

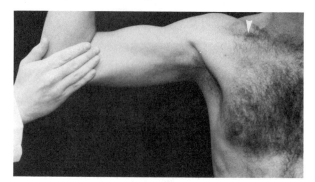

Figure 52

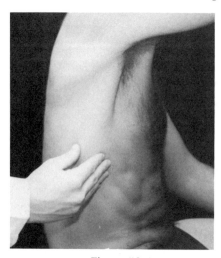

Figure 53

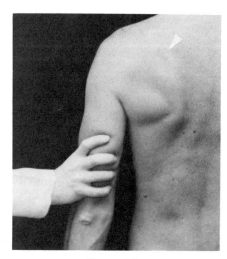

Figure 54

FIG. 51 Adduction of the arm (toward the trunk)

Sternocostal portion of pectoralis major (lateral and medial anterior thoracic nerves, C5–T1)
Teres major (lower subscapular nerve, C5–7)
Latissimus dorsi (thoracodorsal nerve, C6–8)

The arm is slightly flexed at the elbow and abducted approximately 25 degrees away from the trunk; the examiner pushes the arm away from the body (while palpating the pectoralis major) as the patient adducts against resistance.

FIG. 52 Adduction of the horizontally abducted arm

Teres major (lower subscapular nerve, C5–7)
Latissimus dorsi (thoracodorsal nerve, C6–8)
Clavicular and sternocostal portions of pectoralis major (lateral and medial anterior thoracic nerves; clavicular—mainly C5–6; sternocostal—mainly C6–T1)

The patient's forearm is flexed at the elbow and the arm is abducted 90 degrees at the shoulder. The examiner places his hand below the elbow and the patient adducts against resistance. Contraction of the pectoralis major is best tested by having the patient bring the elbow forward.

FIG. 53 The cough test

Latissimus dorsi (thoracodorsal nerve, C6–8)

The examiner grasps the muscle near the inferior angle of the scapula and contraction can be felt when the patient coughs.

FIG. 54 Initial abduction (elevation) of the upper arm: 0 to 15 degrees

Supraspinatus (suprascapular nerve, C5–6)
Deltoid (axillary nerve, C5–6)
Lower two-thirds of trapezius (CN XI and C3–4)—aids in fixing scapula

The patient's arm is fully adducted and the patient abducts the upper arm against resistance. Note: after the initial 10 to 15 degrees of abduction, the deltoid is the primary muscle of abduction.

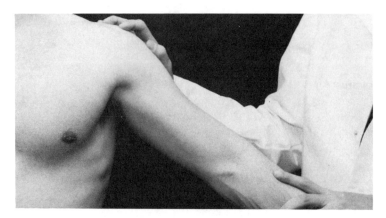

Figure 55

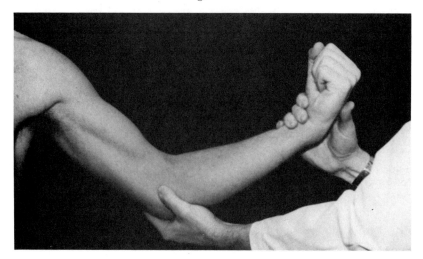

Figure 56

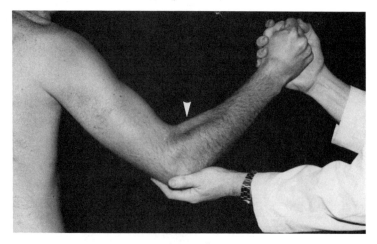

Figure 57

FIG. 55 Abduction (elevation) of the upper arm: 15 to 90 degrees

Deltoid (axillary nerve, C5–6)

The patient abducts the arm roughly 45 degrees and then attempts further abduction against resistance.

FIG. 56 Flexion of the forearm at the elbow

Biceps (musculocutaneous nerve, C5–6)
Brachialis (musculocutaneous nerve, C5–6)
Brachioradialis (radial nerve, C5–6)
Pronator teres (median nerve, C6–7)

The forearm is fully supinated and flexed 90 degrees at the elbow. The patient attempts further flexion against resistance.

FIG. 57 Test of brachioradialis function

Brachioradialis (radial nerve, C5–6)

The forearm is midway between supination and pronation, and flexed 90 degrees at the elbow. The patient attempts further flexion against resistance. Contraction of the brachioradialis is seen, for example, when a glass is steadied as it is brought towards the lips.

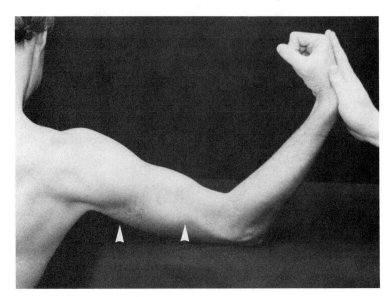

Figure 58

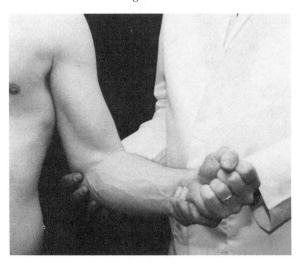

Figure 59

FIG. 58 Extension of the forearm at the elbow

Triceps (radial nerve, C6–8)
Anconeus (radial nerve, C7–8)

The arm is slightly abducted (to eliminate the influence of gravity) and the forearm is slightly flexed. The patient extends the forearm against resistance.

FIG. 59 Forearm supination

Biceps (musculocutaneous nerve, C5–6)
Supinator (posterior interosseous nerve, C6–7)
Brachioradialis (radial nerve, C5–6)

The forearm is flexed 90 degrees at the elbow and slightly pronated; the elbow is placed against the body. The patient tries to supinate the forearm against resistance.

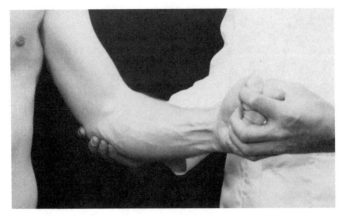

Figure 60

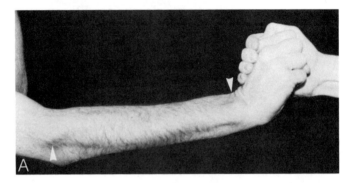

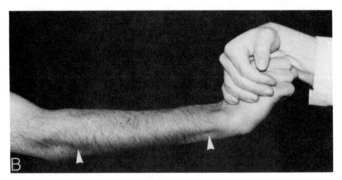

Figure 61

FIG. 60 Forearm pronation

Pronator teres (median nerve, C6–7)
Pronator quadratus (anterior interosseous nerve, C7–T1)
Palmaris longus (median nerve, C7–T1)
Flexor carpi radialis (median nerve, C6–7)
(The last two muscles are only active in forearm pronation when resistance is
applied)

The forearm is flexed 90 degrees at the elbow with the arm slightly abducted
(externally rotated) at the shoulder; the elbow is placed against the body. The
patient tries to pronate the forearm against resistance.

FIG. 61 Extension (dorsiflexion) of the hand at the wrist

Extensor carpi radialis longus (radial nerve, C5–6)
Extensor carpi radialis brevis (radial nerve, C5–6)
Extensor carpi ulnaris (posterior interosseous nerve, C7–8)
Extensor digitorum (posterior interosseous nerve, C7–8)

The forearm is flexed at the elbow (to a roughly 135 degree angle with arm) and
the extensor carpi radialis longus and brevis (**A**) and extensor carpi ulnaris (**B**)
are tested. In testing these muscles it is best to watch the muscle bellies contract
and to palpate the tendons.

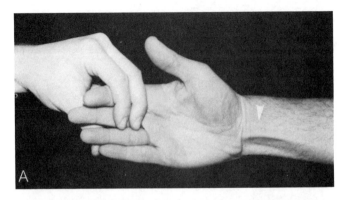

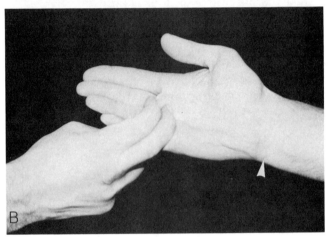

Figure 62

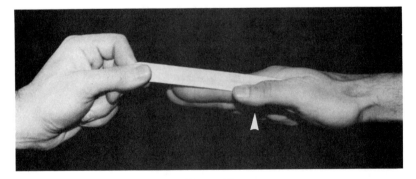

Figure 63

FIG. 62 Palmar flexion of the hand at the wrist

Flexor carpi radialis (median nerve, C6–7)
Flexor carpi ulnaris (ulnar nerve, C7–T1)
Abductor pollicis longus (posterior interosseous nerve, C7–8)
Palmaris longus (median nerve, C7–T1)

To test the flexor carpi radialis (**A**), the examiner places his second and third digits across the patient's fingers and the patient tries to flex the hand at the wrist. The tendon of the flexor carpi radialis is lateral to that of the palmaris longus. To test the flexor carpi ulnaris (**B**), the examiner places his second and third digits across the fourth and fifth fingers and the patient tries to flex the hand at the wrist.

FIG. 63 Ulnar adduction (in the plane of the palm)

Adductor pollicis (deep branch of ulnar nerve, C8–T1)
Extensor pollicis longus (posterior interosseous nerve, C7–8)
Opponens pollicis (lateral terminal branch of the median nerve, C8–T1)
Flexor pollicis longus (anterior interosseous branch of the median nerve, C7–8)
Flexor pollicis brevis (superficial head supplied by the lateral terminal branch of
   the median nerve; deep head by the deep branch of the ulnar nerve; C8–T1)

This action is tested by asking the patient to maintain a piece of paper (or tongue blade) between the radial border of the hand and the thumb while the examiner attempts to remove it.

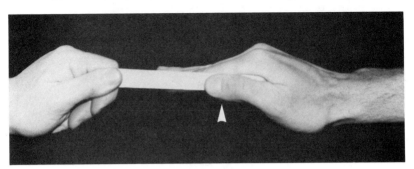

Figure 64

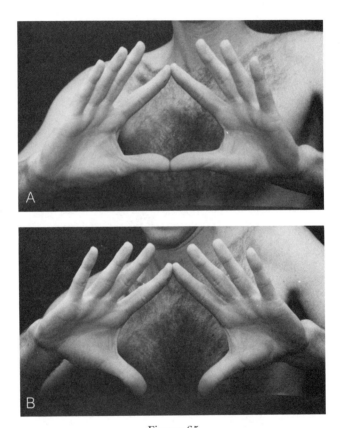

Figure 65

FIG. 64 Palmar adduction of the thumb (in the plane at a right angle to the palm)

First interossei—dorsal and palmar (deep branch of the ulnar nerve, C8–T1)
Extensor pollicis longus (posterior interosseous nerve, C7–8)

This action is tested by asking the patient to maintain a piece of paper or a tongue blade between the thumb and the hand as shown in the figure.

Note: With complete ulnar nerve lesions, both ulnar and palmar adduction of the thumb can be performed by the extensor pollicis brevis.

FIG. 65 Radial abduction of the thumb (in the plane of the palm)

Abductor pollicis longus, extensor pollicis brevis and longus (posterior interosseous nerve, C7–8)
Abductor pollicis brevis (lateral terminal branch of the median nerve, C8–T1)

Have the patient bring the hands in front of him with the palms facing the examiner, then ask him to bring the tips of the index fingers together, and then to separate the thumbs and index fingers as in the figure.

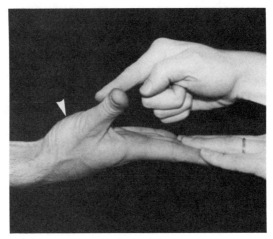

Figure 66

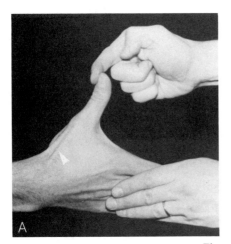
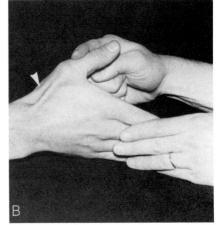

Figure 67

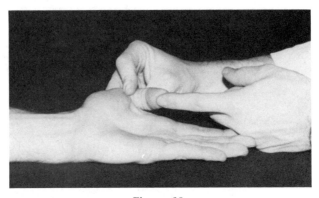

Figure 68

FIG. 66 Palmar abduction of the thumb (in the plane at a right angle to the palm)

Abductor pollicis brevis (lateral terminal branch of the median nerve, C8–T1)
Flexor pollicis brevis (lateral terminal branch of the median nerve, C8–T1)
Opponens pollicis (lateral terminal branch of the median nerve, C8–T1)
Abductor pollicis longus (posterior interosseous nerve, C7–8)

This action is tested by asking the patient to move the thumb away from the other fingers at a right angle to the plane of the palm.

FIG. 67 Thumb extension

Extensor pollicis longus—extension of the distal (and less so, the proximal) phalanx (posterior interosseous nerve, C7–8)
Extensor pollicis brevis—extension of the proximal phalanx (posterior interosseous nerve, C7–8)

The ulnar border of the patient's hand is placed at a 90 degree angle to the table; begin with the thumb in palmar abduction. Extension of the distal (**A**) and proximal (**B**) phalanges can be tested separately, as shown.

FIG. 68 Thumb flexion

Flexor pollicis longus—flexion of the proximal and distal phalanx (anterior interosseous branch of median nerve, C7–8)
Flexor pollicis brevis—flexion of the proximal phalanx (superficial head— lateral terminal branch of median nerve; deep head—deep branch of ulnar nerve; C8–T1)
Abductor pollicis brevis—flexion of the proximal phalanx (lateral terminal branch of median nerve, C8–T1)
Adductor pollicis—flexion of the proximal phalanx (deep branch of ulnar nerve, C8–T1)

With the thumb in palmar adduction and the proximal phalanx immobilized by the examiner, flexion of the distal phalanx can be tested, and allows assessment of the flexor pollicis longus in isolation. To test flexion at the proximal phalanx, the thumb is maintained in palmar adduction and the metacarpal is immobilized.

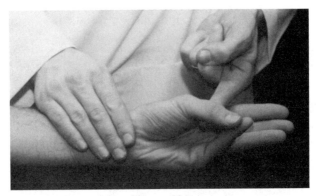

Figure 69

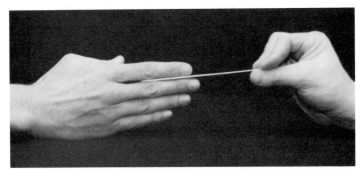

Figure 70

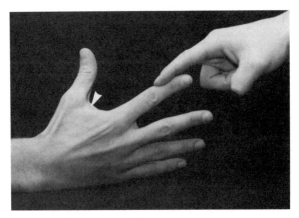

Figure 71

FIG. 69 Thumb opposition

Opponens pollicis (lateral terminal branch of the median nerve, C8–T1)
Flexor pollicis brevis (deep head; deep branch of the ulnar nerve, C8–T1)
Abductor pollicis brevis (lateral terminal branch of median nerve, C8–T1)

The palmar surface of the thumb is placed so that it touches the tip of the fifth finger, and the patient attempts to maintain this position against resistance.

FIG. 70 Finger adduction (except the thumb)

Palmar interossei (deep branch of ulnar nerve, C8–T1)

This movement is tested by asking the patient to bring the extended fingers close together and try to keep a piece of paper (or a tongue blade) between them while the examiner attempts to remove it. Care should be taken to exclude participation of the thumb or flexion of the fingers.

FIG. 71 Finger abduction (except the thumb)

Dorsal interossei (deep branch of the ulnar nerve; rarely, the first dorsal
  interosseous is supplied by the median nerve; C8–T1)
Abductor digiti minimi—abducts the fifth digit (deep branch of the ulnar nerve,
  C8–T1)

The patient is asked to extend and spread apart all the fingers and resist the examiner's efforts to push them together.

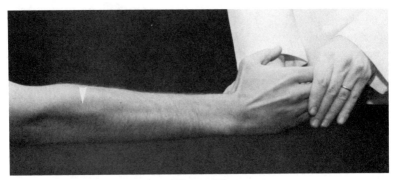

Figure 72

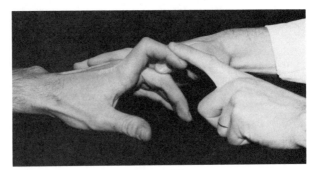

Figure 73

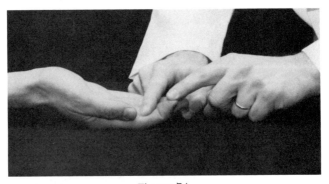

Figure 74

FIG. 72 Finger extension at the metacarpophalangeal joint (except the thumb)

Extensor digitorum (posterior interosseous nerve, C7–8)
Extensor indicis—extends the second digit (posterior interosseous nerve, C7–8)
Extensor digit quinti—extends the fifth digit (posterior interosseous nerve, C7–8)

The proximal and distal interphalangeal joints are flexed and the metacarpophalangeal joint is extended against resistance.

FIG. 73 Finger extension at the proximal interphalangeal joint of the index finger

First lumbrical (median nerve, C8–T1)

Note: The first and second lumbricals are supplied by the median nerve (C8–T1); the third and fourth lumbricals are supplied by the deep branch of the ulnar nerve (C8–T1).

Palmar and dorsal interossei (deep branch of ulnar nerve, C8–T1)

The metacarpophalangeal joint of the index finger is extended while the proximal interphalangeal joint is slightly flexed; the patient extends the proximal interphalangeal joint against resistance.

FIG. 74 Finger flexion at the distal phalanges (except the thumb)

Flexor digitorum profundus (supply to the second and third digits—anterior interosseous nerve (median), C7–8; supply to the fourth and fifth digits—ulnar nerve, C7–8)

The examiner immobilizes the middle phalanx while the patient flexes the distal phalanx against resistance.

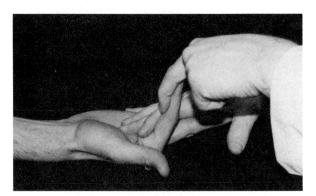

Figure 75

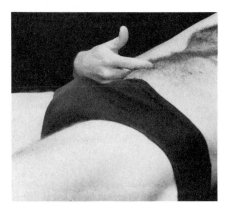

Figure 76

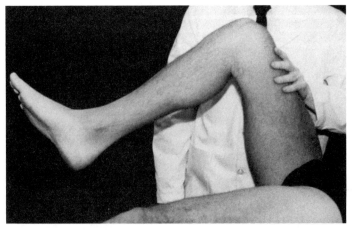

Figure 77

FIG. 75 Finger flexion at the middle phalanges (except the thumb)

Flexor digitorum superficialis (median nerve, C7–T1)

The examiner immobilizes the proximal phalanx while the patient flexes the middle phalanx. The action of the flexor digitorum profundus can only be eliminated by keeping the distal phalanx flaccid, which is difficult.

INSPIRATION

Diaphragm (phrenic nerve, C3–5)
Intercostal muscles (segmental supply by intercostal nerves, T1–T12)

Observe spontaneous respiration and deep breathing. Decreased excursion of the chest wall on one side (best appreciated by observing the movement of the costal margin) with inspiration may result from unilateral phrenic nerve lesions, upper motor neuron lesions, or local pathology. Respiratory status can be monitored by vital capacity measurements and by asking the patient to take a deep breath, exhale fully, and then count aloud without inspiring again.

Note: When respiration appears to be entirely abdominal, consider weakness of the intercostal muscles (segmental supply by the intercostal nerves, T1–12) This possibility is supported by the finding of retraction of the intercostal spaces during inspiration.

FIG. 76 Test of abdominal muscles—Beevor's sign

Rectus abdominis (intercostal nerves, T5–12)
Internal oblique (intercostal nerves, T7–12; iliohypogastric nerve, L1)
External oblique (intercostal nerves, T7–12; iliohypogastric nerve, L1)

The patient lies supine and attempts to raise his head against resistance. The examiner should place a finger at the level of the umbilicus and note deviation of the umbilicus. Upward deviation is a positive *Beevor's sign;* it reflects weakness of the lower abdominal muscles and often results from spinal cord compression at the midthoracic level. Unilateral deviation of the umbilicus may also be observed; it may result from a lesion of several intercostal nerves (or roots), for example, by a paraspinal mass.

FIG. 77 Hip flexion

Iliopsoas (psoas—L1–3; iliacus—femoral nerve, L1–3)

In order to best eliminate the action of supporting muscles and test the iliopsoas, the leg should be flexed 90 degrees at the knee and the thigh should be flexed 90 degrees at the hip. The patient is then asked to flex against resistance.

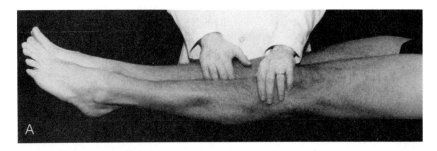

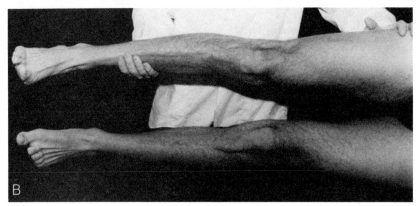

Figure 78

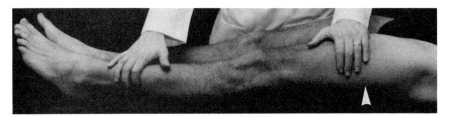

Figure 79

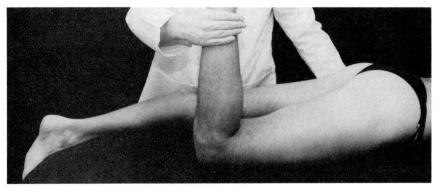

Figure 80

FIG. 78 Adduction of the thigh

Adductors—magnus, brevis, longus (obturator nerve, L2–4)
Gluteus maximus—lower fibers (interior gluteal nerve, L5–S2)

First, the examiner tests both legs simultaneously to compare relative strength **(A)**. Then, each leg should be tested separately **(B)**.

FIG. 79 Thigh abduction

Gluteus medius (superior gluteal nerve, L4–S1)
Tensor fasciae latae (superior gluteal nerve, L4–S1)
Gluteus minimus (superior gluteal nerve, L4–S1)

In the supine position, the patient attempts to abduct his leg against resistance.

Note: this action has an important L5 innervation and may be helpful in differentiating weakness of distal L5 innervated muscles (e.g., extensor hallucis longus, peronei) caused by proximal and distal lesions.

FIG. 80 Medial (internal) rotation of the leg

Gluteus medius (superior gluteal nerve, L4–S1)
Tensor fasciae latae (superior gluteal nerve, L4–S1)
Gluteus minimus (superior gluteal nerve, L4–S1)

In the prone position with the leg flexed 90 degrees at the knee, the patient attempts to turn the lower leg laterally against resistance.

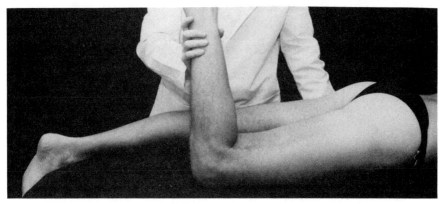

Figure 81

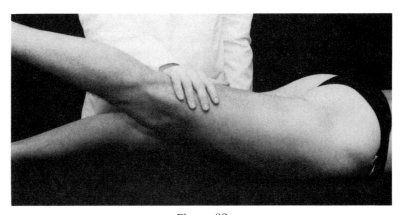

Figure 82

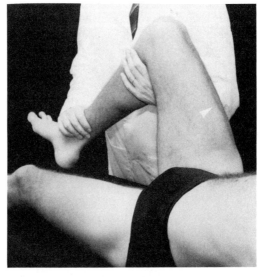

Figure 83

FIG. 81 Lateral (external) rotation of the leg

Gluteus maximus—lower fibers (inferior gluteal nerve, L4–S2)
Obturator internus (nerve to obturator internus, L5–S1)
Gemelli—superior & inferior (superior—nerve to the obturator internus, L5–S1; inferior—nerve to the quadratus femoris, L5–S1)

In the prone position with the leg flexed 90 degrees at the knee, the patient attempts to turn the lower leg medially (lateral rotation) against resistance.

FIG. 82 Hip extension

Gluteus maximus (inferior gluteal nerve, L5–S2)
Gluteus medius—posterior fibers (superior gluteal nerve, L4–S1)

In the prone position with the leg slightly flexed at the knee, the patient lifts his leg and attempts to hold the leg off the table against resistance. One of the examiner's hands should palpate the contracting muscle.

FIG. 83 Knee extension

Quadratus femoris (rectus femoris, vastus lateralis, vastus intermedius, vastus medialis) (femoral nerve, L2–4)

In the supine position with the leg flexed 90 degrees at the knee and the thigh flexed, the patient attempts to extend the knee against resistance.

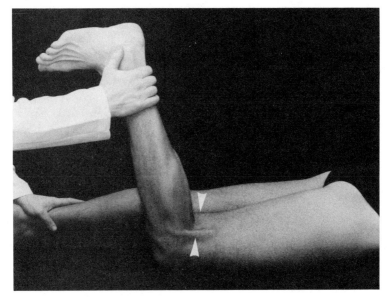

Figure 84

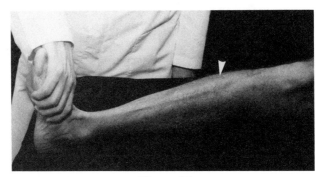

Figure 85

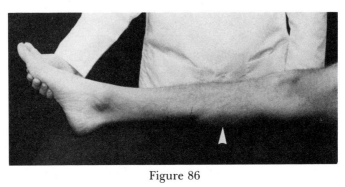

Figure 86

FIG. 84 Knee flexion

Hamstrings—biceps femoris/semitendinosus/semimembranosus (sciatic nerve, L5–S2)

This is best tested with the patient in the prone position (if the patient is supine, flexion of the thigh may be mistaken for flexion of the knee); the lower leg is flexed at the knee and the patient attempts to maintain this position against resistance.

FIG. 85 Foot dorsiflexion

Tibialis anterior (deep peroneal nerve, L4–5)
Extensor digitorum longus (deep peroneal nerve, L5–S1)
Extensor hallucis longus (deep peroneal nerve, L5–S1)

The patient dorsiflexes the foot against resistance.

FIG. 86 Plantar flexion of the foot

Gastrocnemius (tibial nerve, S1–2)
Soleus (tibial nerve, S1–2)
Tibialis posterior (tibial nerve, L4–5)
Flexor digitorum longus (tibial nerve, L5–S2)
Flexor hallucis longus (tibial nerve, L5–S2)

The patient attempts to maintain plantar flexion of the foot against resistance; the examiner should palpate the contracting gastrocnemius.

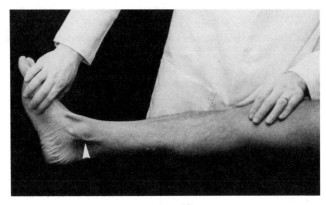

Figure 87

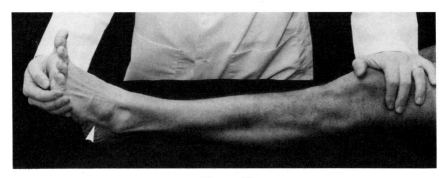

Figure 88

FIG. 87 Inversion of the foot

Tibialis posterior (tibial nerve, L4–5)
Tibialis anterior (deep peroneal nerve, L4–5)
Flexor digitorum longus (tibial nerve, L5–S2)
Flexor hallucis longus (tibial nerve, L5–S2)
Extensor hallucis longus (deep peroneal nerve, L5–S1)

The patient inverts (turns inward) the foot and attempts to maintain this position against resistance; the examiner should palpate the tendons of the tibialis posterior and anterior.

FIG. 88 Eversion of the foot

Peroneus longus (superficial peroneal nerve, L5–S1)
Peroneus brevis (superficial peroneal nerve, L5–S1)
Extensor digitorum longus (deep peroneal nerve, L5–S1)

The patient everts (turns outward) his foot and attempts to maintain this position against resistance; the tendons of the peronei should be palpated.

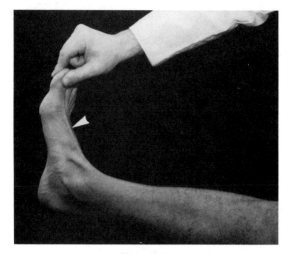

Figure 89

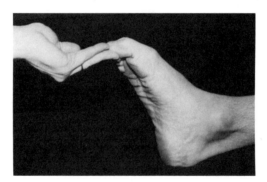

Figure 90

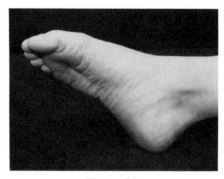

Figure 91

FIG. 89 Toe dorsiflexion (extension)

Extensor hallucis longus—extension of the great toe (deep peroneal nerve, L5–S1)
Extensor digitorum longus—extends the second to fifth toes (deep peroneal nerve, L5–S1)
Extensor digitorum brevis—extends the first to fourth toes (deep peroneal nerve, L5–S1)

The patient extends the great toe against resistance; the examiner should palpate the tendon of the extensor hallucis longus and the belly of the extensor digitorum brevis.

FIG. 90 Plantar flexion of the toes

Flexor hallucis longus—flexes all the toes (tibial nerve, L5–S2)
Flexor hallucis brevis—flexes all the toes (medial plantar nerve (tibial nerve branch), S1–2)
Flexor digiti quinti brevis—flexes the fifth toe (superficial branch of the lateral plantar nerve (tibial nerve branch), S1–2)

The patient flexes the great toe (or other toes) against resistance.

FIG. 91 Cupping of the sole of the foot

Small muscles of the foot (medial and lateral plantar nerves (branches of the tibial nerve), S1–2)

The patient is asked to cup the sole of the foot.

SENSORY EXAMINATION

I. General principles

   A. First ask the patient to outline the area of sensory abnormality.
   B. Be sure to distinguish weakness (which may be perceived as "numbness") from sensory loss.
   C. The importance of repeated examinations cannot be overemphasized. *The most important exam is often the second one.*
   D. When there is an area of decreased sensitivity, begin testing sensation there and move toward the normal area. With areas of hypersensitivity, begin in the normal area.
   E. When testing pin sensation, alternate sharp and dull stimuli and ask patient to respond as soon as possible.
   F. Intermittently ask patient to point to the exact area of stimulation (topognosis).
   G. Loss of sensation to pinprick is often less than loss of light touch or temperature sensation.
   H. Temperature sensation testing may give more consistent evidence of sensory loss than pinprick.
   I. When sensory loss includes deep pain (e.g., to pinching of the Achilles tendon), it suggests complete nerve injury.
   J. Keep in mind the possibility of sensory inattention caused by parietal lobe lesions.
   K. Two-point discrimination is a sensitive method to compare the two sides. Normal values are

Lips	2–3 mm
Back	40–50 mm
Palms	8–15 mm
Dorsum of hands	20–30 mm
Dorsum of feet	30–40 mm
Fingertips	3–5 mm
Dorsum of fingers	4–6 mm
Shins	30–40 mm

II. Important patterns of sensory loss:

   A. Compression of peripheral nerves or nerve roots is more likely to affect large fibers (which conduct joint position and vibratory sensation) than small fibers (pain and temperature sensation).
   B. There may be loss of vibratory sensation without loss of proprioception in subacute combined degeneration, syringomyelia, and occasionally in multiple sclerosis; the opposite pattern of sensory loss may occur with parietal lobe lesions.
   C. A classic pattern is dissociated sensory loss of central cord lesions— loss of pain/temperature sensation with preservation of position/ vibratory sensation.

D. Plexus lesions—if in the proximal plexus, plexus lesions simulate multiple root lesions; if in the distal plexus, they simulate multiple peripheral nerve lesions.

REFLEX EXAMINATION

1. The stimulus used to elicit a reflex should be a threshold one; i.e., no greater than necessary. The muscle to be stimulated should be in a state of slight contraction. Grade the individual reflex and always test and compare the two sides of the body in symmetric positions.
2. Reinforcement maneuvers can help elicit reflexes that are apparently absent or difficult to elicit. Since stretching of a muscle by the percussion is the stimulus necessary for the deep reflex, reinforcement is best accomplished by *slight* voluntary contraction of the muscle tested. For example, a patient might push the lower leg slightly forward while the examiner opposes the movement and simultaneously strikes the patellar tendon.
3. Any stimulus that produces brisk muscle stretch—direct or indirect—can evoke the muscle's stretch reflex. Thus, percussion of a bone or other firm part of a limb or the trunk can stimulate muscles at a distance and evoke an unexpected muscle stretch reflex; that is the basis for "reflex spread." In states of organic or functional reflex hyperirritability reflexes are more easily elicited at a distance because the overall tonus and, thus, muscle stretch are enhanced. Therefore, in a patient with brisk reflexes, a tap on the radius may initiate reflex contraction in biceps, triceps, and finger flexors and extensors as well as brachioradialis. The limb moves in the direction of the stronger muscle, and thus the result is forearm flexion. This phenomenon can explain "paradoxical" and "inverted" reflexes. When the triceps reflex arc is damaged, a blow to the elbow may inadvertently stretch the flexors of the arm which then reflexively contract normally, unopposed by reflex triceps contraction, producing the "paradoxical" reflex. Disease of cord segments C5 and C6 interrupts the brachioradialis reflex arc, but radial percussion may produce reflex contraction of the triceps and finger flexors, an "inverted" reflex.
4. Tendon or bone tapping may evoke spinal automatisms. Thus, tapping the Achilles tendon may produce dorsiflexion rather than plantar flexion of the foot.
5. Cutaneous reflexes cannot be elicited in an anesthetic field. They usually recover before deep tendon reflexes. Unusual responses may occur if motor function recovery lags behind sensory recovery.

For example, tibial nerve injury may impair plantar flexion, but if sensation has recovered, stroking the foot can result in dorsiflexion of the toes, a "peripheral" Babinski response. Cutaneous reflexes may be abolished with corticospinal tract lesions.

6. Reflex deficits usually appear at the time of injury and persist after other functions are restored.

7. Reflex dysfunction provides no index of lesion severity. Partial nerve interruption may impair reflexes. Also, reflexes may be preserved despite impairment in other muscles supplied by nerves or roots that subserve the reflex. For example, the triceps reflex may be elicited if the long head of the triceps is spared.

8. In primary muscle disease (e.g., myopathy or myositis) reflexes remain until muscle contraction itself is absent.

9. Reflexes may be increased early in peripheral nerve lesions, perhaps because of irritability of the afferent nerves.

10. Severe contracture producing joint immobility may result in *apparent* loss of reflexes; careful observation reveals the presence of muscle contraction. *Palpation may be required to detect slight reflex contraction.*

11. Reflexes may be graded as follows:

    0   not elictable
    1   elicited with reinforcement
    2   normal
    3   brisk
    4   clonus (unsustained)
    5   sustained clonus

AUTONOMIC NERVOUS SYSTEM EXAMINATION

I. Anatomy and physiology—see Table 8, p. 53.

II. Clinical features of autonomic disorders

A. Sympathetic efferents to cutaneous blood vessels and sweat glands travel in the peripheral nerves (PN); PN lesions cause characteristic changes:

1. *Vasomotor changes.* The initial phase (roughly 2 weeks) is marked by increased skin temperature and rosy color followed by decreased temperature, mottling (pallor and cyanosis), and edema. Prolonged vasomotor changes are common with partial PN lesions and PN lesions accompanied by causalgic pain.

2. *Sweat deficit.* With complete PN lesions, the area of anhydrosis is often greater than that of hypesthesia. With partial PN

lesions, excessive sweating may reflect regeneration or irritative phenomena.

3. *Trophic changes.* Trophic changes occur especially in hands and feet, and are often accompanied by irritation (e.g., repeated minor trauma secondary to decreased sensation). Initially they appear as indentations of skin; chronically as inelastic, smooth, shiny (atrophic) skin. With partial PN lesions (especially of the median and ulnar nerve), eczema or hyperkeratosis may develop. Fingernails may become clubbed, develop transverse white stripes, or become brittle or thick. Alopecia or hypertrichosis (especially on the forearm) may occur.

III. Tests of autonomic function

A. *Pupillary functions.* Note the size, shape, and location of the pupils. Anisocoria (inequality of pupil size) due to oculomotor lesions is most prominent in bright light, whereas that due to Horner's syndrome (HS) is most prominent in dim light. Look for slight ptosis or anhidrosis in association with miosis (HS).

1. Parasympathetic dysfunction causes mydriasis with loss of light reflex and accommodation. Denervation hypersensitivity (present after roughly 2 weeks) can be demonstrated by pupillary constriction with 2.5% methacholine eye drops (normally there is no response).

2. Sympathetic dysfunction causes miosis, which is often accompanied by mild ptosis and anhidrosis in HS. Central lesions of sympathetic pathways affect sweating over the entire hemibody, whereas peripheral lesions (i.e., distal to the superior cervical ganglion) may affect sweating on the face. Pre- and postganglionic lesions may be differentiated by cocaine (4%) and hydroxyamphetamine (1%) eye drops given sequentially to both eyes (it may take several hours for cocaine to exert its maximum effect, and one must wait 48 hours for its effect to dissipate before administering hydroxyamphetamine).

RESPONSE	COCAINE 4%	OH-AMPHETAMINE 1%
Normal	Mydriasis	Mydriasis
With preganglionic lesion	Slight mydriasis	Mydriasis
With postganglionic lesion	No response	No response

B. Lacrimation—deficit may follow pre-geniculate ganglion facial nerve lesion.

1. Reflex tearing may be tested by having the patient smell noxious stimuli (e.g., ammonia) or by irritating the cornea (afferent

limb—trigeminal nerve; efferent limb—facial nerve to ptery-gopalatine ganglion, postganglionic fibers pass through maxillary nerve).

2. *Schirmer test.* Relative tear production may be quantified by applying a strip of filter paper to each medial conjunctiva.

C. *Salivation.* A deficit in salivation may occur in pre- or post-geniculate ganglion facial nerve lesions. Reflex secretion follows sucking on a lemon or lime and may be observed by inspection of the submaxillary duct (afferent limb—facial and glossopharyngeal nerves; efferent limbs—facial and glossopharyngeal nerves, via submandibular and otic ganglia, respectively).

D. *Heart rate.* For the following tests involving heart rate (HR) (except for the carotid sinus reflex), it should be remembered that HR response (i.e., HR variation) is greater in young subjects.

1. *Valsalva maneuver.* The normal ratio of maximal tachycardia (phase II; during forced expiration) to maximal bradycardia (phase IV; during recovery) is greater than 1.5. Test by having the patient give a strong forced expiration against a closed glottis for 15 to 20 sec; monitor HR with EKG.

2. *Beat-to-beat variation in HR.* Normally, with deep breathing at a rate of 6 to 8/min, there will be at least a 15 beat/min difference variation in HR (measure R–R intervals with EKG).

3. *Carotid sinus massage.* Gentle rubbing of the carotid bifurcation on one side may cause reflex slowing of HR. This reflex may be absent in normal individuals and overactive in the elderly. Complications include arrhythmias which may be hemodynamically significant and possibly stroke resulting from dislodged thromboemboli.

4. *Hyperventilation.* Normally, deep breathing at a rate of 30/min for 20 to 25 sec will increase the HR by more than 12 beats/min.

5. *Postural change.* Normally, going from the supine to the upright position will increase HR by 10 to 20 beats/min.

E. Blood pressure (sympathetic).

1. Postural change. Normally, going from the supine to the upright position does not decrease mean BP (systolic pressure may fall slightly); in the elderly there may be a 10 mmHg fall in mean BP.

2. *Cold pressor test.* Place entire hand in ice water (4°C) for 1 minute and monitor BP every 20 to 30 sec. The normal response is a greater than 15 mmHg rise in systolic and a greater than 10 mmHg rise in diastolic pressure.

F. *GI motility*. GI motility is deficient with parasympathetic lesions. Document the deficiency with barium study of esophageal, gastric, and small bowel function.

G. *Sweating*. Sweating can be assessed by lightly rubbing the fingers across the skin to detect the presence of moisture; compare an area with the same area the contralateral and with adjacent areas. (Axillary sweating may be preserved despite autonomic insufficiency). More specific tests are as follows:

1. *Starch-iodine test*. Paint the patient with a solution of iodine (15 g), castor oil (100 ml), and dilute alcohol (900 ml), allow it to dry, and then dust with starch. Sweat will cause the starch to turn blue-black.
2. *Thermoregulatory sweating*. Increase ambient temperature and look for areas of diminished sweating. Rectal temperature must increase at least 0.5°C and there must be at least a 30 min latent period.
3. *Axonal reflex*. Inject 0.1 ml of 1:10,000 acetylcholine intradermally and check for sweating 1 to 2 min later; sweating will be absent with peripheral nerve lesions.

H. *Vasomotor and trophic changes that accompany reflex sympathetic dystrophy*. Test axonal reflex by intradermal injection of 0.1 ml 1:1,000 histamine; flare is absent with complete peripheral nerve lesions.

I. *Anal sphincter*. (External muscle has somatic and internal has parasympathetic innervation.) Test the integrity of the anal sphincter during rectal exam by noting tone and asking patient to bear down.

J. *Urinary bladder*. Depending on symptoms and associated findings, it may be appropriate to obtain a urinalysis/culture, perform a careful rectal exam with attention to the prostate gland, measure postvoiding residual volume, or obtain a cystometrogram.

SELECTED
CLINICAL
PROBLEMS

PERIPHERAL NEUROPATHY WITH SYSTEMIC DISEASE

TABLE 10. Peripheral Neuropathy with Systemic Disease

SYSTEMIC DISEASE	PREDOMINANT TYPE OF NEUROPATHY[a]	ONSET AND COURSE[a]	PATHOLOGY[a]
Metabolic disorders			
Uremia	Sensory (sensorimotor)	Chronic (acute)	AD (SD)
Porphyria	Motor	Acute	AD
Hypoglycemia	Motor	Chronic	AD
Endocrine disorders			
Diabetes mellitus	Sensorimotor–autonomic[b,c]	Chronic (subacute)	AD (SD)
Hypothyroidism	Sensory[b]	Chronic	AD
Acromegaly	Sensory[b]	Chronic	AD
Malignancies and reticuloses			
Carcinoma	Sensory, sensorimotor	Subacute or chronic (acute)	AD (SD in acute sensorimotor and relapsing type)
Lymphoma	Sensorimotor	Acute, subacute or chronic	AD, (SD in relapsing type)
Chronic lymphocytic leukemia	Sensorimotor	Acute (subacute)	AD
Polycythemia vera	Sensory	Chronic	AD
Deficiency states			
Vitamin B_{12}	Sensory	Chronic	AD
Thiamine	Sensorimotor	Chronic	AD
Folic acid	Sensory	Chronic	AD
Vitamin E	Sensory	Chronic	AD

Paraproteinemias and dysproteinemias			
Primary amyloidosis	Sensory (sensorimotor–autonomic)[b]	Chronic (subacute)	Amyloid deposition
Multiple myeloma	Sensorimotor (motor or sensory)	Chronic	AD
Cryoglobulinemia	Sensorimotor	Chronic	AD
Macroglobulinemia	Sensorimotor	Subacute or chronic (acute)	AD (SD)
Monoclonal gammopathy			
IgA	Sensorimotor, motor	Chronic	AD
IgG	Sensorimotor	Chronic	AD (SD)
IgM	Sensorimotor	Chronic	SD
Connective tissue disorders			
Systemic lupus erythematosus	Sensorimotor[b,c]	Chronic (subacute)	AD
Rheumatoid arthritis	Sensory (sensorimotor)[b,c]	Chronic (subacute)	AD
Miscellaneous			
Chronic liver disease	Sensory (sensorimotor)	Chronic	SD
Primary biliary cirrhosis	Sensory	Chronic	AD
Viral hepatitis	Sensory, sensorimotor	Acute	SD
Adult celiac disease	Sensorimotor	Chronic	AD
Chronic obstructive pulmonary disease	Sensory (sensorimotor)	Chronic	AD
Sarcoidosis	Sensorimotor, sensory or motor	Acute or chronic	AD

AD = axonal degeneration; SD = segmental demyelination.
[a] Words in parentheses indicate less common types.
[b] Entrapment neuropathies may also occur.
[c] Mononeuritis or mononeuritis mulitplex may also occur.
(Reprinted with modification by permission of the publisher from Asbury AK, Gilliatt RW (eds.): Peripheral Nerve Disorders. London: Butterworths (Publishers) Ltd. 1984, p. 93.)

PAINFUL SENSORY NEUROPATHIES

TABLE 11. Painful Sensory Neuropathies[a]

Focal neuropathies
Diabetes mellitus
Compression
Polyarteritis nodosa
Herpes zoster (pre- and postherpetic neuralgia)
Brachial plexus neuropathy

Polyneuropathies—described as deep persistent ache or superficial stinging/burning
Amyloidosis
Diabetes mellitus
Multiple myeloma
Acute idiopathic polyneuritis (Guillain-Barré syndrome)—often back pain early
Carcinoma
Cryoglobulinemia
Hypothyroidism
Alcohol
Thiamine deficiency
Uremia
Insulinoma
Fabry's disease
Tangier disease
Dominantly inherited sensory neuropathy

[a] Common in neuropathies affecting small myelinated and unmyelinated fibers, and secondary to ischemia of nervi nervorum.

HYSTERIA

Neurologic signs and symptoms should be diagnosed as hysterical only with great caution; follow-up studies at academic centers reveal a misdiagnosis rate of 25–50%. Most errors are failure to identify peripheral nerve, spinal cord, muscle, connective tissue, skeletal, and partial seizure disorders. *The presence of functional disease does not preclude the coexistence of organic disease—they often coexist.* Misdiagnosis of psychiatric illness as neurologic is also common and may result in dangerous and costly studies and treatments while effective therapy is not given. The most common conversion symptoms are paralysis, syncope, sensory loss, seizures, visual loss, and movement disorders. The choice of symptom is influenced by previous lesion/symptom, dominant side (more commonly affected), and iatrogenic suggestion.

The diagnosis of hysteria is not made simply by excluding organic causes or by the paucity of neurologic signs in the face of prominent symptoms; positive evidence must be sought (such as findings not consistent with neuroanatomy/physiology). The patient should be observed carefully during spontaneous behavior and when they are unaware of another's presence. Psychologic factors should be considered—mood ("how have your spirits been lately?" should be part of every history), life events, indifference, secondary gain.

HYSTERICAL PARALYSIS
Hysterical paralysis often fluctuates with repeated exams and suggestion; the examiner often senses a lack of effort; contraction of antagonist muscles can be seen/palpated or revealed by sudden release or increase in resistance; muscles that are "paralyzed" when tested as prime movers may function normally as synergists. Some tests to detect these signs are as follows:

1. The examiner abducts the arm to 90 degrees and suddenly removes support—the "paralyzed" limb briefly maintains position.
2. While testing the biceps or triceps or brachioradialis, the examiner suddenly changes from resisting to assisting the muscle—the arm returns towards the original position (due to the antagonist).
3. With the wrist dropped the patient can make a strong fist (which requires the wrist extensors as synergists).
4. With the patient supine the "paralyzed" arm is dropped so that gravity should make it strike the face, but it consistently misses.
5. Thigh adduction test—while adducting the "normal" leg, the examiner rests his hand on the "paralyzed" thigh to detect contraction.
6. Hoover test—the patient flexes the "normal" thigh while supine, and the examiner's other hand rests under the "paralyzed" leg to detect reciprocal extension.
7. Gait—the examiner may observe lack of circumduction and wear on the shoetoe (spastic); presence of inert dragging of the leg which is assisted by arm, wild reeling from side to side without effort to maintain equilibrium, improvement in unsteadiness when the patient is distracted (e.g., testing rapid alternating movements of fingers).

HYSTERICAL SENSORY DISTURBANCES
Hysterical sensory disturbances often fluctuate with repeated exams and suggestion, tend to be extensive, and involve all modalities. There is a sharp demarcation between normal and abnormal areas which corresponds to surface landmarks such as joints but not to dermatomal or nerve supply, and which splits along the midline precisely. Hysterical sensory disturbances may be detected by tests such as the following:

1. Apply vibration to a point on the insensitive side from which bone conduction would transmit the signal to the normal side (e.g., the forehead)—a hysterical patient will deny feeling the vibration.

2. Test the patient's ability to touch finger to nose or heel to shin with the eyes closed to assess proprioception.
3. In a patient with complete anesthesia, test with a mildly noxious stimulus during sleep.
4. Pain—initially, one must always accept the patient's description of pain as real and organic, even if it is bizarre and obviously elaborated. But consider depression and a somatization disorder.

MYOFASCIAL PAIN SYNDROMES

Myofascial pain (MP) is a common cause of musculoskeletal pain but is frequently overlooked and improperly treated. Recognizing it requires knowledge of specific patterns of referred pain by individual muscles. MP arises from activation/irritation of a trigger point (TP) in a muscle or adjacent fascia. A TP is a focus of hypersensitivity in the muscle or fascia which causes pain spontaneously (active TP) or only with direct palpation (latent TP).

HISTORY
The examiner should obtain details of the movements and activities associated with onset or recurrence of pain; onset may be abrupt or gradual. Ask patient to localize the point of maximal pain and to describe the distribution of pain. Loss of sensation or strength or the presence of paresthesia are not characteristic of MP.

PHYSICAL EXAMINATION
Palpation of affected muscles usually reveals rope-like taut bands. Passive stretch or voluntary contraction of muscles with TPs may cause local or referred pain. Restricted range of motion may result from taut bands. An important objective sign is the local twitch response—brief (usually less than 1 sec) contraction of a local group of muscle fibers following a brisk, snapping palpation of the TP; this response strongly suggestive of a diagnosis of MP.

NERVE ENTRAPMENT SYNDROMES

NEUROLOGIC THORACIC OUTLET SYNDROMES

Neurologic thoracic outlet syndromes have a low incidence; there is a strong female predominance (up to 9×). They occur between ages 10 and 80 years (peak incidence between ages 20 and 40 years).

☐ **SYMPTOMS.** Intermittent ache that may be accompanied by paresthesia in medial arm and forearm is typical at onset but is usually mild (patients consult a physician an average of 5 years after the onset of sensory symptoms and 2 years after the onset of motor symptoms). Weakness and wasting of hand muscles (restricted to or most prominent in the thenar eminence) is common, whereas motor forearm involvement (most marked in flexors) occurs in approximately 25% of cases. Variable sensory loss, most often on the medial forearm, may occur. Unilateral involvement is the rule. Vascular changes are infrequent and Adson's maneuver is of doubtful significance. The cause of the syndrome is usually compression of the lower brachial plexus by a fibrous band from the transverse process of C7 to the rudimentary first rib.

DIGITAL NERVE ENTRAPMENT IN THE HAND

Entrapment of the digital nerve in the hand is uncommon; acute trauma causes pain, tenderness, swelling, and numbness, whereas chronic lesions (mass, trauma) cause sensory loss, pain, or paresthesias of the hemidigit. Trauma, occupational factors (e.g., bowling), arthritis/osteophytes, and benign tumors are the main causes.

SUPRASCAPULAR NERVE ENTRAPMENT

Suprascapular nerve entrapment is uncommon; it presents with shoulder pain and weakness of shoulder abduction (due to supra- and infraspinatus involvement) without sensory loss. There is often tenderness over the suprascapular notch (the site of compression). The etiology is traumatic or idiopathic.

MEDIAN NERVE ENTRAPMENT

Carpal Tunnel Syndrome

In carpal tunnel syndrome the site of compression is the carpal tunnel (bounded by the transverse carpal ligament above, the bony carpus laterally and below, and containing the median nerve and flexor tendons).

□ **INCIDENCE.** The syndrome is common; females predominate (3×); 60% of cases present between 40 and 60 years of age.

□ **SYMPTOMS.** The syndrome presents with intermittent numbness, pain, and paresthesia in median distribution. The symptoms are nocturnal or accompany prolonged wrist flexion. They may be relieved by shaking the hand. Later, symptoms are more persistent; sensory symptoms are greater than motor symptoms. Pain may occur in any part of the upper extremity.

□ **SIGNS.** Characteristic signs are absent in the early stages. Sensory loss (maximal on the volar tips of the second and third digits) is greater than motor loss (thenar atropy, weakness of the abductor pollicis brevis and the opponens pollicis). Tinel's sign and Phalen's test are positive.

□ **ETIOLOGY.** The cause may be tenosynovitis (idiopathic most common), rheumatoid arthritis, amyloidosis, infection, gout, sarcoid, trauma, tumors, pregnancy, acromegaly, hypothyroidism.

Anterior Interosseous Nerve (Branch of Median Nerve) Syndrome

Anterior interosseous nerve syndrome presents with elbow/proximal forearm pain. There is weakness of flexion of the interphalangeal joint of the thumb (flexor pollicis longus) and of distal interphalangeal joints of the second and third digits (flexor digitorum profundus). Trauma is the most common cause; the syndrome also may be caused by compression by fibrous bands and anomalous tendons (roughly 10 cm distal to elbow).

Pronator Syndrome

□ **COMPRESSION OF THE MEDIAN NERVE NEAR THE ELBOW.** Pronator syndrome caused by compression at this site presents with pain and "fatigue/tiredness" of the proximal forearm; symptoms often follow activity with repeated elbow movements. Proximal forearm tenderness is common; motor and sensory signs are variable and usually mild. Compression between the two heads of the pronator teres may result from trauma, hypertrophy, or fibrous bands.

□ **COMPRESSION OF THE MEDIAN NERVE AT THE PROXIMAL HUMERUS.** Pronator syndrome caused by compression at this site is uncommon; it may present with paresthesia in the median nerve distribution on elbow extension, or with weakness. It is usually caused by a ligament connecting the supracondylar bony spur (often palpable) to the medial epicondyle of the humerus.

ULNAR NERVE ENTRAPMENT

□ **COMPRESSION AT THE ELBOW.** Ulnar nerve entrapment at the elbow is common; it usually presents with numbness and tingling of the fourth and fifth digits and medial palm; there may be elbow pain that radiates distally. Sensory loss is most common in the distal two phalanges of the fifth finger (autonomous ulnar supply). Froment's sign, worsening penmanship, mild clawing and loss of dexterity, and hypothenar atrophy may occur. Compression occurs in the condylar groove (superficial, lateral to the medial epicondyle of humerus) or in the cubital tunnel. Trauma is a common cause at the former site, and excessive elbow flexion at the latter site.

□ **COMPRESSION AT GUYON'S CANAL.** Ulnar nerve entrapment at Guyon's canal (ulnar tunnel; bounded by the transverse and volar carpal ligaments, the pisiform, and the hook of the hamate) at the wrist usually causes pure motor neuropathy affecting ulnar-supplied intrinsics, and spares the hypothenar muscles. Sensory loss over the volar surface of the fourth and fifth digits and wrist pain may occur. Compression at this site is caused by trauma, ganglion, ulnar artery lesions, and occupational factors (e.g., bicycling).

RADIAL NERVE ENTRAPMENT

□ **COMPRESSION IN THE AXILLA.** Radial nerve entrapment in the axilla is uncommon; it results in weakness of the triceps and other radial innervated muscles, and may result from crutches or trauma.

□ **COMPRESSION IN THE MID-ARM.** The mid-arm is the most common site of radial entrapment; there is wrist drop with normal triceps strength; sensory loss is variable and if present is often limited to a patch on the dorsum of the hand between the first and second digits. The site of compression is the spiral groove or intermuscular septum. Compression may result from improper positioning of arm during sleep (especially while intoxicated—"Saturday night palsy"), tourniquets, and general anesthesia.

□ **COMPRESSION IMMEDIATEDLY DISTAL TO ELBOW.** Radial nerve entrapment just distal to the elbow ("posterior interosseus nerve motor syndrome") causes pure motor deficit—weakness of thumb and finger extensors with relative sparing of wrist extension. It may be accompanied by transient pain in the elbow/proximal forearm. It is usually due to compression by lipomas, ganglia, and fibromas. It has a role as a cause of "resistant tennis elbow"; the presence of maximal tenderness over the posterior interosseous nerve as it passes through the supinator, and increased pain with active supination, help distinguish it from the more common lateral epicondylitis (maximal tenderness over the lateral epicondyle).

□ COMPRESSION AT THE WRIST. Superficial radial nerve lesions at or proximal to the wrist may cause sensory loss and paresthesia in radial distribution; sympathetic dystrophy may result. They usually result from tight bracelets, wristbands, casts, and laceration/fracture; they may be iatrogenic (for example, caused by IV shunts for dialysis).

SCIATIC NERVE ENTRAPMENT

Sciatic nerve entrapment is uncommon; it rarely causes complete palsy. Sensory and motor findings are variable; pain often mimics sciatica but spares the lower back. Compression of the nerve as it passes through the piriformis ("piriformis syndrome") causes buttock pain radiating distally without neurologic signs. Other causes include coma, anesthesia, or prolonged sitting in unusual positions; hematomas; fibrous bands; and lipomas. Pelvic and rectal examinations are essential.

COMMON PERONEAL NERVE ENTRAPMENT

Common peroneal nerve entrapment is common; cachectic patients and those on analgesics are predisposed to develop it; it usually presents as painless foot drop in which sensory loss is absent or mild (in either superficial or deep peroneal distribution). The nerve is usually compressed as it winds laterally around the neck of the fibula and passes through the superficial head of the peroneus longus (fibular canal). Causes include prolonged sitting with legs crossed or squatting or kneeling, trauma, tight casts or stockings, or surgery in the lithotomy position.

TARSAL TUNNEL SYNDROME

Tarsal tunnel syndrome presents with pain in the sole, often with burning paresthesias and often worse at night. Sensory loss is variable, but if present, occurs over the plantar surface of the foot. Tinel's sign may be elicited over the tarsal tunnel (posterior and inferior to the medial malleolus). Motor findings are often absent or mild; weakness of plantar flexion of the lateral toes is the most often found. The tarsal tunnel runs just below the medial malleolus and also carries the posterior tibial artery and the tendons of the flexor digitorum longus, flexor hallucis longus, and tibialis posterior. Trauma and improper footwear are the most common causes; thrombophlebitis and tenosynovitis may also be causes.

LATERAL FEMORAL CUTANEOUS NERVE ENTRAPMENT—MERALGIA PARESTHETICA

Lateral femoral cutaneous nerve entrapment presents with paresthesias of the upper lateral thigh; it is often precipitated by light touch (e.g., of clothing) over affected skin, by tapping the inguinal ligament just below the anterior iliac spine (the usual site of compression), by prolonged upright position or extension of the leg at the hip. A patch of sensory loss is often present in the center of this nerve's distribution. Motor changes are absent. Entrapment often results from tight garments and is more common with obesity, diabetes, and pregnancy.